New Tools for Psychoanalysis

Bringing together the findings from psychoanalysts across the globe, this book introduces and describes the research practices utilised by the Working Parties that were created by the European Psychoanalytical Federation and later supported by the International Psychoanalytical Association.

The book opens with a discussion of the epistemology of research in psychoanalysis, then the various Working Parties describe their methodology and findings, and finally, in the last chapter, an assessment is made of what contributions this oxygenating movement has made to psychoanalysis. It examines topics including individual and group work, supervision, clinical interpretation, erotic transference and psychosomatics, and contains contributions from many distinguished analysts.

Providing a wealth of information on the place of research in evaluating new clinical methods and tools, this book is key reading for psychoanalysts both in practice and in training.

Ruggero Levy is a psychoanalyst, full member and training analyst of the Porto Alegre Psychoanalytical Society (SPPA); former chair of the IPA Working Parties Committee (2017–2021); former IPA board member (2011–2013 and 2013–2021); gave the keynote paper at the IPA Congress in 2017; and is former president of the SPPA.

Bernard Reith is a training and supervising analyst and former president of the Swiss Society of Psychoanalysis; regional editor for Europe of the *International Journal of Psychoanalysis*; former co-chair for Europe of the IPA Working Parties Committee (2017–2021) and chair (2021–2023); and former chair of the EPF Working Party on Initiating Psychoanalysis (2005–2016).

Agustina Fernández is a psychoanalyst, full member and training analyst of the Argentine Psychoanalytic Association (APA); co-chair for Latin America of the IPA Working Parties Committee (2017–2021 and 2021–2023); chair of the LA Working Party on Specificity of Psychoanalysis Today (2021–2023); former co-chair of FEPAL Working Parties Commission 2012–2014 and former chair (2014–2016).

Leopoldo Bleger left Argentina in 1976, where he trained as a medical doctor and psychiatrist, and has lived in Paris since. He is a "supervisor analyst" of the French Association. He is a member of the EPF WP on Specificity of the Psychoanalytic Treatment Today and was general secretary of the European Federation (2012–2016) and president of his society (2017–2019).

Nancy Kulish is a faculty member and training and supervising analyst of the Michigan Psychoanalytic Institute and adjunct professor, Department of Psychiatry, Wayne State Medical School. She is a member of the IPA Working Parties Committee and gave the Plenary Panel address on Sexuality at the International Psychoanalytic Congress in Mexico City, 2011.

Marie G. Rudden is training and supervising analyst of the American Psychoanalytic Association; co-chair of the North American Comparative Clinical Methods Working Party; associate editor, *International Journal of Applied Psychoanalytic Studies*; on the North American Editorial Board, *International Journal of Psychoanalysis*; and co-author, *Psychodynamic Treatment of Depression* (first and second editions), APA.

Inés Bayona Villegas is a psychoanalyst and full member of the Colombian Psychoanalytic Society; former IPA chair for Latin America of the Interregional Encyclopedia and Dictionary of Psychoanalysis (2019–2022) and author of *Dear Candidate* (2021).

'*New Tools for Psychoanalysis* is a remarkable book that describes the history, development and the different forms of one of the most creative achievements of psychoanalysis supported and stimulated by IPA: the working parties. The editors and contributors are the analysts who developed and currently chair the working parties; each chapter is a true masterclass richly illustrated with clinical material. I strongly recommend the reading of this comprehensive and scholarly-written new book, which shows the vitality of contemporary psychoanalysis. As someone who took part in the collective effort to develop this fascinating new psychoanalytic tool, I am sure that the readers will enjoy the symbiosis of scientific method and aesthetic experience that the book provides.'

Cláudio Laks Eizirik, *former president of the IPA*

'The Working Parties were and are the most courageous, innovative and creative experiment of mutual knowledge and theoretical–clinical fertilisation in the psychoanalytic community. By periodically confronting live clinical material provided by analysts from all over the world, groups of geographically and culturally heterogenous colleagues have been able to evolve individually and at the same time have contributed to substantial collective progress in our scientific field. This book, written by yesterday's and today's protagonists of this wonderful adventure, is absolutely recommendable as a fundamental text for understanding contemporary psychoanalysis.'

Stefano Bolognini, *former president of the IPA, founder of the Inter-Regional Encyclopedic Dictionary of Psychoanalysis*

'Twenty years ago, the European Psychoanalytic Federation initiated a series of working parties to study psychoanalysis psychoanalytically. They were to focus on psychoanalytic data such as case presentations and employ psychoanalytic methods such as free associative listening. The project has since been taken over by the International Psychoanalytic Association, has expanded around the world, and has become a dominant theme in the intellectual life of the profession. This volume, the creation of 31 leading psychoanalysts, presents a valuable summary of ten of these working parties and provides the foundation for the next stage of inquiry in psychoanalysis.'

Robert Michels, MD, *Walsh McDermott University professor of Medicine and Psychiatry, Weill Cornell Medicine; president, Board of Directors,* The Psychoanalytic Quarterly; *former joint editor-in-chief,* The International Journal of Psychoanalysis

The *New Library of Psychoanalysis* is published by Routledge Mental Health in association with the *Institute of Psychoanalysis*, London.
The purpose of the book series is:

- to advance and disseminate ideas in psychoanalysis amongst those working in psychoanalysis, psychotherapy and related fields
- to facilitate a greater and more widespread appreciation of psychoanalysis in the general book-reading public
- to provide a forum for increasing mutual understanding between psychoanalysts and those in other disciplines
- to facilitate communication between different traditions and cultures within psychoanalysis, making some of the work of continental and other non-English speaking analysts more readily available to English-speaking readers, and increasing the interchange of ideas between British and American analysts.

The *New Library of Psychoanalysis* published its first book in 1987 under the editorship of David Tuckett, who was followed by Elizabeth Bott Spillius, Susan Budd, Dana Birksted-Breen and Alessandra Lemma. The Editors, including the current Editor, Anne Patterson, have been assisted by a considerable number of Associate Editors and readers from a range of countries and psychoanalytic traditions. The present Associate Editors are Susanne Calice, Katalin Lanczi and Anna Streeruwitz.

Under the guidance of Foreign Rights Editors, a considerable number of the *New Library* books have been published abroad, particularly in Brazil, Germany, France, Italy, Peru, Spain and Japan. The *New Library of Psychoanalysis* has also translated and published several books by continental psychoanalysts and plans to continue the policy of publishing books that express as clearly as possible a variety of psychoanalytic points of view. The *New Library of Psychoanalysis* has published books representing all three schools of thought in British psychoanalysis, including a particularly important work edited by Pearl King and Riccardo Steiner, *'The Freud-Klein*

Controversies 1941–45', expounding the intellectual and organisational controversies that developed in the British psychoanalytical Society between Kleinian, Viennese and 'middle group' analysts during the Second World War.

The *New Library of Psychoanalysis* aims for excellence in psychoanalytic publishing. Submitted manuscripts are rigorously peer-reviewed in order to ensure high standards of scholarship, clinical communications, and writing.

For a full list of all the titles in the New Library of Psychoanalysis main series as well as both the New Library of Psychoanalysis 'Teaching Series' and 'Beyond the Couch' subseries, please visit the Routledge website.

New Tools for Psychoanalysis

Clinical Investigation and Psychoanalytic
Training in the Working Parties

Edited by Ruggero Levy, Bernard Reith,
Marie G. Rudden, Agustina Fernández,
Nancy Kulish, Leopoldo Bleger
and Inés Bayona Villegas

Routledge
Taylor & Francis Group

LONDON AND NEW YORK

Designed cover image: MartinStr © pixabay

First published 2024
by Routledge
4 Park Square, Milton Park, Abingdon, Oxon OX14 4RN

and by Routledge
605 Third Avenue, New York, NY 10158

Routledge is an imprint of the Taylor & Francis Group, an informa business

© 2024 selection and editorial matter, Ruggero Levy, Bernard Reith, Marie G. Rudden, Agustina Fernández, Nancy Kulish, Leopoldo Bleger and Inés Bayona Villegas; individual chapters, the contributors

The right of Ruggero Levy, Bernard Reith, Marie G. Rudden, Agustina Fernández, Nancy Kulish, Leopoldo Bleger and Inés Bayona Villegas to be identified as the authors of the editorial material, and of the authors for their individual chapters, has been asserted in accordance with sections 77 and 78 of the Copyright, Designs and Patents Act 1988.

All rights reserved. No part of this book may be reprinted or reproduced or utilised in any form or by any electronic, mechanical, or other means, now known or hereafter invented, including photocopying and recording, or in any information storage or retrieval system, without permission in writing from the publishers.

Trademark notice: Product or corporate names may be trademarks or registered trademarks, and are used only for identification and explanation without intent to infringe.

British Library Cataloguing-in-Publication Data
A catalogue record for this book is available from the British Library

Library of Congress Cataloging-in-Publication Data
Names: Levy, Ruggero, editor.
Title: New tools for psychoanalysis : clinical investigation
   and psychoanalytic training in the working parties / edited by
   Ruggero Levy [and 6 others]
Other titles: New library of psychoanalysis
Description: Abingdon, Oxon : New York, NY: Routledge, 2024. |
   Series: New library of psychoanalysis | Includes bibliographical
   references and index.
Identifiers: LCCN 2023037499 (print) | LCCN 2023037500 (ebook)
Subjects: MESH: Fédération européenne de psychanalyse. | International
   Psycho-Analytical Association. | Psychoanalysis—methods |
   Research Design | Psychoanalytic Therapy—methods | Societies |
   Congresses as Topic
Classification: LCC RC506 .N494 2024 (print) | LCC RC506 (ebook) |
   NLM WM 460 | DDC 616.89/17072—dc23/eng/20231121
LC record available at https://lccn.loc.gov/2023037499
LC ebook record available at https://lccn.loc.gov/2023037500

ISBN: 978-1-032-65627-4 (hbk)
ISBN: 978-1-032-65628-1 (pbk)
ISBN: 978-1-032-65631-1 (ebk)

DOI: 10.4324/9781032656311

Typeset in Bembo
by Apex CoVantage, LLC

We dedicate this book to all those who actively participated in the various Working Parties held all over the world.

Contents

Contents

Presentation

The Working Parties are tools created by the European Psychoanalytic Federation about 20 years ago with the purpose of creating spaces for dialogue, reflection, and psychoanalytic research. They are groups of clinical psychoanalysts that have developed specific methodologies to investigate a certain clinical issue of psychoanalysis or of psychoanalytic training.

The IPA in 2016 created the IPA Working Parties Committee with the aim of stimulating the scientific production of these groups from their findings in their clinical workshops, because we understand that these clinical research groups are very rich tools for the scientific development of psychoanalysis. The Working Parties Committee also intends to create bridges of dialogue between the various Working Parties so they don't remain working in isolation. To achieve this goal, we held several panels and symposia in partnership with EPF, FEPAL, NAPSAAC, and APSAA, and this book is the result of all this work.

We want to thank the IPA and the regional federations for their support, and especially all the WP groups that joined our project. Thank you all!

INTRODUCTION

New Tools for Psychoanalysis[1]

The IPA Working Parties Committee members

The Working Parties, together with the related endeavours described in this book, occupy a space between scientific exploration and intersubjective dialogue, sharing characteristics of both disciplines. Sigmund Freud always thought of psychoanalysis as a scientific endeavour. He hoped for scientific validation of his field but recognized that there would be a long and circuitous road ahead. Because he saw psychoanalysis as an observational science, he understood that much more work would be needed before attaining well-grounded descriptions and theories. As he wrote in *An Autobiographical Study* (Freud, 1925, pp. 57–58):

> Clear basic concepts and sharply drawn definitions are only possible in the mental sciences in so far as the latter seek to fit a region of facts into the frame of a logical system. In the natural sciences, of which psychology is one, such clear-cut and general concepts are superfluous and indeed impossible. Zoology and Botany did not start from correct and adequate definitions of animal and plant. . . . Physics itself . . . would never have made any advance if it had had to wait until its concepts of matter, force, gravitation, and so on, had reached the desirable degree of clarity and precision. . . . Psycho-analysis was constantly reproached for its incompleteness and insufficiencies; though it is plain that a science based upon observation has no alternative but to work out its findings piecemeal and to solve its problems step by step.

DOI: 10.4324/9781032656311-1

Freud the psychoanalyst was careful to point out that science doesn't always advance in the way one imagines and that certainty is an illusory ideal, but his ambition that psychoanalysis should work "step by step" to be recognized as a scientific discipline remains transparent.

The Working Parties arose from the recognition that one of these essential "steps" involves better communication between psychoanalysts about how they understand their work and the clinical observations in which it is grounded. The inherently subjective nature of psychoanalytic work means that this communication involves sharing and comparing subjectivities. Intersubjective sharing can be emotionally challenging, so that methods must be found to support it; and yet such methods must not block the spontaneous creativity of the exchange, which permits better communal insight into the unconscious realities being studied.

As we will see, various methods have been found to sustain this intersubjective work, but their underlying spirit resembles that of approaches described in contemporary educational science, political science, and philosophy. In these fields, as in psychoanalysis, facts are important, but equally so are individual perceptions of them, which may be erroneous, but which may also reveal hitherto important neglected or unexpected truths. Working through these perceptions cannot be done merely through logical reasoning, or dialectic: it also requires intersubjective dialogue. Here is how one contemporary philosopher, Dmitri Nikulin, states the issue in his *Dialectic and Dialogue* (Nikulin, 2010, pp. 132–133):

> Oral dialogue . . . is more precise than an established argument that can meticulously gather and reproduce hundreds of steps in the correct order of reasoning. . . . Oral speech is precise not literally (according to the "letter") but in terms of its meaning . . . which . . . is subject to revision over and over in any oral dialogue and throughout the generations of its tradition. Since the very "life of the mind" consists in debate and dialogical discussion, which is both a starting point and a point of destination, there is no need for an ultimate or definitely established speech that will become the standard of reference. . . . Yet it is the renewable and always seemingly different oral logos that is universal, for by belonging to everyone who participates . . . it can always continue unwrapping, clarifying, and rendering more precise an idea or personal other.

Nikulin recognizes the value of science and other forms of rigorous exploration and argumentation, but he locates them within an essential, unending cultural and intersubjective process of dialogue allowing a richer and more precise perception of reality. The psychoanalytic reader will easily see how his description applies also to ongoing work in the psychoanalytic community. Moreover, Nikulin's concept of the "personal other," which appears at the end of the quotation, resembles something that all psychoanalysts can recognize: the descriptively and dynamically unconscious internal stranger in oneself, of whose existence one is unaware, and who can only be revealed in the context of encounters with others – as in the psychoanalytic relationship, in the unplanned and unexpected exchanges of intersubjective or inter-analytic dialogue, and, as we will describe, in the peer group work of Working Party workshops.

Before going more deeply into our subject, we will use the experience of Dr A. to illustrate something of both aspects, scientific research and creative dialogue, of the Working Party endeavour. This took place nearly 20 years ago, near the beginning of the Working Party movement.

Rolling Up Our Shirtsleeves

Dr A. travelled with some trepidation to a far-away country to present session material at a Working Party clinical workshop. His first surprise came when he entered the room. He was a bit intimidated to recognize two well-known, internationally admired senior analysts, but there were also colleagues of all ages he didn't know, including some more junior analysts like himself. Everyone was sitting in good humour and in disarray around a big table, shirtsleeves rolled up (it was a hot day), with no obvious hierarchical positions except for that of the moderator sitting at one end. Dr A. had read the workshop instructions beforehand so he could have expected this, but it nevertheless came across as unusual.

The next surprise dawned on him slowly as the work progressed. Dr A. had been anxious to show that he was working well in a difficult analysis, but during their lively exchanges he realized this wasn't what interested them. The group just assumed that he was working analytically but was curious to understand *how* he worked and *why* he worked as he did. Whether he worked "well" or not wasn't the issue: the question was more whether he worked the way he thought he did and, if not, what other dynamics could be involved.

The procedures of this workshop involved paying close attention to the analyst's interventions, where they occurred in the session and why, what he hoped to achieve with them, why he worded them as he did, and so on. This was where something really astonishing happened. Dr A. believed that here-and-now interpretative work in the transference was the key to helping his paranoid patient to see how she defended against her cumulative traumatic experiences. But one workshop member detected a different pattern in his work. He pointed out that in the session they were looking at, Dr A.'s first intervention linked the patient's associations to the setting; his next intervention was a word aiming to facilitate the associative process; next, he linked some of the patient's associations; later, he interpreted the patient's emotional and phantasy experience with the analyst; only then, after further associations on her part, did he give a complete transference interpretation, which involved a reconstruction related to the patient's infantile experience and phantasy. Interestingly, during the last part of the session he worked in the exact reverse order, ending with another comment about the setting. It was as if he thought that he should work with her carefully until they could enter the central theme of the session and then ease her way back out before leaving each other for the day.

Dr A. hadn't realized this at all. He and the workshop looked again at all the sessions he had presented, and they found the same pattern every time. He had no explicit psychoanalytic theory to explain this way of working. Something implicit or unconscious was at stake. In the ensuing workshop discussion, he thought that the patient's paranoid transference might induce him to be particularly cautious with her. Based on the contents of the session and her childhood history, however, he also wondered whether he might be working like a surgeon in an emergency unit, carefully opening level by level to intervene where the problem was, and then carefully stitching layer by layer on his way back out. He left the workshop thinking that he might be sharing the patient's paranoid theory about her distress, as something dangerous to be taken out rather than something to be integrated. His own infantile sexual phantasies could also be at work, as well as a phantasy of being a better object tenderly picking up a starving baby from her cot, feeding her, and gingerly putting her back to sleep.

Thinking in Cases

Dr A.'s experience is what the Working Parties are all about. Psychoanalysts come together, not to tell each other how the work "should" be done because, as Freud states cogently in the quotation earlier, we cannot be sure that we have the right kind of knowledge for that, but instead to help each other to explore their field and their position in it, and to deepen their understanding of both.

Such work is done through "thinking in cases" (Forrester, 2017). Close examination of single cases does not aim to insert them into a predefined "logical system" using "clear basic concepts and sharply drawn definitions." Rather, what is learned from each new case points to potentially significant themes, patterns, or lines of thought that might be useful for understanding the field or suggest directions for future exploration. The aim is to empower thinking, not to find sure knowledge. Ideas about general patterns are the tentative outcome of such exploration, not its starting point, and are always modifiable by the study of new cases. In psychoanalytic terms, hoping for certainty would be a regression to a phantasy of having recovered a lost object, instead of keeping the mind open to life, desire, incompleteness, and the unknown (Moss, 2018).

The clinical workshop encountered a telling example of how psychoanalytic technique can be influenced by the countertransference and by the analyst's own transference, as well as, perhaps, an unconscious sense of what might be the best technique. We know that this happens, but it is a boon to be able to discuss it openly and through shared examination of detailed process material. In this specific workshop procedure, detailed attention to the structure and timing of the analyst's interventions seems to have accompanied and stimulated rather than hampered the free-associative work. As for Dr A., he encountered a "personal other" (Nikulin, 2010), an aspect of himself that he hadn't seen and which the dialogue with his colleagues helped him to discover. He came out of the workshop with many new questions about himself and about psychoanalysis and with enlivened, opened perspectives on his work with this patient.

We are thus in a field which has frontiers both with science, as we will discuss more in depth later in this chapter, and with our specifically psychoanalytic work of engaging with the unconscious. The dialogue that takes place between these frontiers is based on a foundation of free-associative inter-analytic group work, although many Working Parties and related efforts combine it with additional procedures, which will be described in each of the following chapters, and whose aim is not to restrict the field but to open it up even more.

Making It Happen

Such group work, however, requires a setting and a method. It is often deemed most successful when psychoanalysts are brought together who are trained in different psychoanalytic models, although good experiences have also been made with analysts working in the same institute. In all cases, the multiplicity of subjective perspectives widens the scope of the investigation and increases its depth, so long as these groups of analysts are organized around their task of exploring the session material, rather than supervising each other. The latter reaction would be to assume sure knowledge and would close the field. This work of exploration calls for clearly defined group procedures and investigative methods, as well as careful moderating. These components are essential for all Working Party settings, including when the method is based exclusively on free-associative inter-analytic group work. A core team of psychoanalysts is therefore needed to define the Working Party's objectives; develop and refine its methods; organize and moderate the workshops; and, last but not least, compile, explore, and publish the workshop findings. This last task of examining the findings also requires the development of approaches specific to their objectives.

The Working Parties and similar undertakings represented in this book were chosen because they all, each in their own specific way, exemplify this tripod of:

1. Clinical workshops where peer groups of psychoanalysts from diverse orientations study analytic sessions;
2. A defined method;
3. A core team responsible for monitoring the process and working through the results.

As happened with the discovery of the psychoanalytic method, this tripod was not defined from the outset. It was the result of a long and complex development.

Finding New Ways of Working Together

Several converging concerns, which were shared worldwide, led the European Psychoanalytic Federation (EPF) to look for new ways for psychoanalysts to work together and communicate better with each other.

One longstanding concern was the frequent tendency of groups of analysts to revert to supervision when discussing clinical material, instead of exploration. Building on the work of pioneers like Michael Balint (1964) and Didier Anzieu (1999), several European groups had addressed this problem, developing and publishing group methods to promote psychoanalytic work on reports of psychoanalytic sessions. Such groups were centred around Wolfgang Loch (1995) in Germany, Jean-Luc Donnet (2005) in France, and Johan Norman and Bjorn Salomonsson (Norman & Salomonsson, 2005; Salomonsson, 2012) in Sweden.

Another major concern was the difficulty encountered by colleagues trained in different psychoanalytic models to understand each other's work. The inherent dynamic relationships between theory, process, and observation in each model meant that psychoanalysts couldn't be sure whether they understood theoretical concepts in the same way, agreed on their clinical observations, or shared each other's expectations about the psychoanalytic process. It was thought that the models might be so fundamentally different that they could even be incommensurable, i.e., impossible to compare (Bernardi, 1989, 1992; Boesky, 2008). If different models led to different processes and so to different clinical observations, then even the search for experience-near common ground (Wallerstein, 1988, 1990) might be a vain hope (Green, 2005). As a result, frustrated colleagues could end up arguing with each other, trying to explain and justify their preferred models, instead of striving to see the psychoanalytic world from other viewpoints. Effective ways had not yet been found to turn misunderstanding between analysts from different analytic cultures into an opportunity for discovery (Faimberg, 2019; see also Chapter 6 in this book). There were fears that such difficulties could lead to deepening rifts between psychoanalytic models, or on the contrary to a resigned attitude that "anything goes" (Tuckett, 2005).

A third concern was the gradual decline in psychoanalytic practice in many European countries, with fewer candidates in training and fewer ongoing high-frequency psychoanalytic treatments per qualified analyst. Less practice meant less experience and less self-confidence, in a vicious circle. Psychoanalysis was also losing its former standing in academia. The pressure to deliver forms of justification for psychoanalytic theory and practice, going beyond single case studies, was thought to be one aspect of this situation, compounded by the fact that many practising analysts found it difficult to identify with the existing standardized research, or were even opposed to it because they perceived the protocols as antithetical to their work in the consulting room. Perhaps complementary ways could be found to ground psychoanalytic investigation in clinical experience, facilitating the dialogue between psychoanalysts, reinforcing their trust in their specialty, and partially bridging the gap between the traditional psychoanalytic single case reports and other forms of research.

These considerations led the EPF, under the impetus of its then President David Tuckett, to begin working in 2000 on its "Ten-year scientific initiative," which was officially launched in 2003. The aim was to encourage "rigorous and sustained activities, securely backed by evidence, aimed at boosting improved clinical work, improved educational activity, clarification of theoretical positions and understanding of how best to try to diffuse our core discipline in the wider world" (Tuckett, 2000). To implement these objectives, four Working Parties were created as task forces or "think tanks" with the aim "to understand and make transparent what we actually do – in clinical work, in the way we use theory in clinical work and in education" (Tuckett, 2003). The assignments of these Working Parties were expressed in their names: WP on Clinical Issues, WP on Theoretical Issues, WP on Psychoanalytic Training (later renamed WP on Education), and WP on Interface (with universities and other professionals). A list of 12 objectives for the next 10 years was laid out, together with funding for meetings and pre-conference activities and requirements about publication. The IPA contributed financially through its Developing Psychoanalytic Practice and Training program (DPPT), until 2007.

All Working Parties principally worked as follows: an internationally composed core group of people were constantly working on their respective objectives. At the EPF conferences they involved other colleagues, shared their work with them, and obtained feedback and critical comment. The basic idea was to create a constant feedback loop, nourishing a hopefully creative recursive process within a peer-group culture and rebuilding confidence (Tuckett, 2002, 2004). The work of sharing and feedback could be done in smaller groups of analysts, often in clinical workshops, or on a wider scale at scientific panels in EPF and other international psychoanalytic congresses. Many types of studies were set up, which would be too numerous to summarize here. Over time, the active involvement of numerous colleagues in the study process through their participation in clinical workshops to examine clinical material (psychoanalytic sessions, supervision sessions, first interviews, etc.), and the development of methods to do so, became central procedures, leading to the development of the tripod that we have outlined earlier.

Controversies and Elaborations

Quite naturally, this ambitious project generated questions and disagreements as well as enthusiasm. One source of disagreement was the choice of methods for the clinical workshops. Early on, differing preferences led the original Working Party on Clinical Issues to divide into two tracks, which respectively became the Forum on Clinical Issues and the Working Party on Comparative Clinical Methods. The Forum on Clinical Issues, later renamed Listening to Listening (Chapter 6), developed a discussion method based on Haydee Faimberg's psychoanalytic work on "listening to listening" and intergenerational dynamics (Faimberg, 2005, 2019), paying attention to the genealogy of psychoanalytic models and the misunderstandings that can result from listening to each other from different background assumptions.

The Working Party on Comparative Clinical Methods or CCM (Chapter 4; see also Tuckett et al., 2008) was interested in developing a method based on Grounded Theory (Glaser & Strauss, 1967; Bryant & Charmaz, 2007), an approach to qualitative research that was first developed in social science but whose basic principles David Tuckett (1994) proposed could be applied in psychoanalysis as well. The basic insight of Grounded Theory is that the intensive, detailed, and methodological study of single cases can be used to generate hypotheses, which can then be tested using the same disciplined study of new and varied cases, including atypical ones or counterexamples. A reflective approach, considering the influence on the findings of the research process itself, is an integral component of some models of grounded theory (Charmaz, 2006; Charmaz & Bryant, 2011) and could be relevant to psychoanalysis because of the psychoanalyst's and psychoanalytic researcher's inevitable and necessary participation in the perception and construction of analytic data (Reith et al., 2018).

The Working Party on Education launched several major projects (Erlich-Ginor, 2010), one of the most successful and enduring of which was End of Training Evaluation (ETE) (Chapter 2; see also Hinze, 2015). A Working Party on Initiating Psychoanalysis (WPIP) was added in 2004 with a broad mandate to better understand the assessment process and to improve the quality of referrals to psychoanalysis; its main research project concerned the dynamics of first interviews (see Reith et al., 2012, 2018 and Chapter 5). Both ETE and WPIP were influenced by Grounded Theory as a useful complement to their specifically psychoanalytic work.

Others, however, felt that introducing what were perceived as extra-analytic methods would interfere with the psychoanalytic work of free association and evenly suspended attention. The Working Party on the Specificity of Psychoanalytic Treatment Today, later renamed the Working Party on the Specificity of Psychoanalytic Treatment through Inter-analytic Group Work (Specificity: Chapter 3), was set up in 2006 in response to this concern by Evelyne Séchaud, then EPF president, and based its workshop methods exclusively on analytic principles (Frisch et al., 2010), influenced by Norman and Salomonsson (2005), Donnet (2005), and Kaës (2005).

10

Later developments in Europe included the setting up of the Free Clinical Groups in 2010 (Chapter 8) and the Working Party on Psychosomatics in 2012 (Chapter 9). The Working Party on Theoretical Issues chaired by Jorge Canestri was the first to wrap up its work with substantial publications (Canestri, 2008, 2012). Other publications followed, as referenced in this book, or are underway.

The work of each of these groups, as well as that of the new groups that were soon set up in North America and Latin America, can be thought of as occupying different locations in the space bounded by psychoanalysis and the variously structured methods of elucidating its theory and practice.

Alongside the debate about methods, another and perhaps more fundamental source of disagreement arose from the very plan of setting up "rigorous and sustained activities, securely backed by evidence." While this was experienced by some as a welcome liberation from dogma and an opening to look at what psychoanalysts really do, as compared to what they believe they do (Sandler, 1983), it was experienced by others as a "violent" (Frisch et al., 2010) and hegemonic attempt to impose a uniform model of psychoanalysis, which would have denatured and impoverished the field. This fear needed to be heard and taken seriously and led to vigorous and salutary debates. The result was that all groups were stimulated to reflect more deeply on the relationships between background assumptions, chosen methods, ensuing processes, and psychoanalytic relevance for their findings, setting off a creative scientific dialogue that continues today (Glover & Reith, 2021).

As in any other institution or group, these debates in EPF could be quite harsh: there were disagreements, critical positions concerning each other's points of view and, of course, rivalry and anathemas. Some Working Parties and similar efforts were in a certain sense created *against* others.

This should not be surprising: it is also a part of any scientific endeavour, and if we consider the history of the psychoanalytic movement, it is nothing new. Although these battles may have (and sometimes unfortunately did have) destructive consequences, they are also a testimony to the aliveness of the debate and to the dedicated involvement of psychoanalysts in their profession. The various Working Parties and related groups still do not agree on many points. But we may remind our readers that psychoanalysis considers conflict to be at the root of psychic life.

In retrospect, we may think that a hope for consensus underlying the Scientific Initiative may have unwittingly produced this sense of imposition. The idea was to create a shared argumentative field (Bernardi, 2002) and a process of public discourse (Habermas, 1984), which are based on taking differences seriously and understanding them, without requiring agreement. But the hope that this argumentative field could be constructed through the search for a more experience-near clinical "common ground" (Wallerstein, 1990) could indeed be thought of as concealing a search for a unified model of psychoanalysis. This is incompatible with the inherently autopoietic nature of psychoanalytic work, which always creates novel configurations not captured by existing models (Schülein, 2003). As authors like Morin (1982, 2005), Nikulin (2010), and Geverif (2017a, 2017b) have pointed out, the search for consensus or for a Hegelian "synthesis" or "sublation" (*Aufhebung*) can lead to the neglect, rejection, or absorption of differing viewpoints and so to an impoverishment of our ability to perceive and think about the intricacies of the world and the life of the mind. However contradictory or incommensurable, each perspective may allow us to represent a significant aspect of a complex reality. Nikulin's (2010) notion of "allosensus" could be relevant here, referring to the challenging task of maintaining an active interest in viewpoints other than one's own, because they may further the process of discovery. Such an approach is analogous in some ways to our analytic work of being curious about the minds of others, however different they are from our own. As psychoanalysts, we would of course add our self-reflective interest in our own unconscious resistances to such encounters and how they may prevent us from learning more.

We might not be looking for our "common ground" in the right place. It might not be found in a unified theory or technique or even in agreement about our clinical observations, but rather in a shared curiosity for working together psychoanalytically on our differences, and in our interest in good questions rather than our defence of favourite answers. In the field of technique, for example, this would not prevent us from judging that some techniques are not good psychoanalytic practice. But it might allow us to understand different techniques better.

In any event, the Scientific Initiative had a profoundly stimulating impact on the life of the EPF. Attendance at the EPF conferences increased and some members and candidates began to say that they were coming more for the pre-conference workshops than for the traditional main conference. Conference attendees coming from the other IPA regions were quick to bring home their enthusiasm.

Developments in North America, Latin America, and the IPA

The Working Parties Within North America

Abbot A. Bronstein introduced the Working Parties to North America in 2008, with the financial and practical support of the International Psychoanalytic Association, as well as the direct support of Harriet Basseches of the North American Psychoanalytic Confederation (NAPsaC). This represented the first attempt at an IPA-funded project within the entire region, including the Canadian and American Psychoanalytic Associations, as well as the independent group of nationally unaffiliated societies and institutes which had become members of the IPA.

The various working parties were introduced by Bronstein, Jorge Canestri, and David Tuckett of the EPF to a large organizing group in New York in 2008. The North American Comparative Clinical Methods WP quickly formed, headed by Abbot A. Bronstein (see Chapter 4), quickly followed by a Working Party on the Specificity of Psychoanalytic Treatment chaired by Ronnie Shaw (Chapter 3). Gradually, the WP for Initiating Psychoanalysis was formed, headed by Nancy H. Wolf (Chapter 5), as was the End of Training WP led by Nancy Kulish and Marianne Robinson (Chapter 2). Moderators for each Working Party were trained by their European counterparts and remained in contact to varying degrees with the European and eventually with the Latin American groups working within the same overarching methodologies. The North American Specificity WP continued to utilize members of the Paris Group as co-moderators, and to actively discuss each of their individual discussion group meetings with the Paris Group.

During the years of IPA funding, a Steering Committee composed of the Chairs of each NA WP and of original members appointed by the presidents of the regional organizations helped to work out budgetary matters and the mechanics of joint scheduling at the different regional meetings.

These four Working Parties have generated presentations at both regional and IPA meetings, as well as published papers on their research (Ehrlich et al., 2017; Rudden & Bronstein, 2015; Wiener-Margulies, 2014).

The Working Parties in Latin America

Working Party activities were also first introduced to Latin American in 2008, at the Congress of the Latin American Psychoanalytic Federation (FEPAL) in Santiago, and further acquaintance was made in 2009 at the IPA Congress in Chicago. It was in 2010, at the FEPAL Congress in Bogota, that they started their activity in the framework of the Pre-Congress. Three groups were held during this congress. The WP on the Specificity of Psychoanalytic Treatment Today was coordinated by Ruggero Levy with the support of Leopoldo Bleger who came from Europe for this purpose; Haydee Faimberg's Method of Listening to Listening was coordinated by Haydee Faimberg and Cláudio Laks Eizirik; and the WP on Comparative Clinical Methods was coordinated by José Carlos Calich. The Latin American colleagues who subsequently started the WPs in the region, besides having participated in several workshops with the European groups, took care to invite colleagues from Europe to train them in the respective methodologies. Since then, the WPs have had an important and growing presence in the FEPAL Congresses: Sao Paulo (2012), Buenos Aires (2014), Cartagena de Indias (2016), and Lima (2018).

In 2013, a WP Commission was created in the FEPAL, chaired by Agustina Fernández, to coordinate the functioning of the groups in the region. In 2015, the Latin American Project of Working Parties was approved by the FEPAL, with the objective of promoting clinical research, strengthening inter-societal work and inter-regional dialogue among the members of the Federation.

In 2020, since the social isolation due to the COVID 19 pandemic, in Latin America some WP groups carried out their first experiences of online work, with very good results.

In this FEPAL framework, of the Latin American Psychoanalytic Federation, seven models were developed over the years, of which five are currently functioning, alongside the IPA Clinical Observation Committee which will be described later: Education (discontinued in 2017); Faimberg's Method of listening to listening

(Chapter 6); Specificity of Psychoanalytic Treatment Today (Chapter 3); Comparative Clinical Methods (Chapter 4); Microscopy of the Analytic Session (Chapter 7); and Unconscious Theories in the Mind of the Analysts at Work.

In some Latin American institutes, the WPs were introduced to candidates as tools for enhancing their psychoanalytic listening. In many societies they also had a continuous education function, revitalizing psychoanalytic listening and reflection about the method.

Developments in the IPA

The International Psychoanalytical Association (IPA) also expressed interest in this way of working. In 2009, during his first administration as IPA president, Charles Hanly defined his main initiatives based mainly on two committees, on Conceptual Integration and on Clinical Observation. They were conceived as Work Groups that in principle were meant to coexist with the Working Parties that were by now being established in all three IPA regions.

However, even though the IPA administration at that time foresaw an exchange between the Work Groups and the Working Parties, it viewed the latter as belonging to the Regional Federations (EPF, FEPAL, and NAPSAC) and, therefore, under the latter's administrative responsibility. The IPA maintained a fund to support the Working Parties until 2013, but then discontinued this financial support, allocating significant funding only to Clinical Observation until this was reduced in 2021.

At first, and as its name implies, Conceptual Integration was given a mandate to search for an integrated theoretical framework for psychoanalysis, but this was soon recognized as unrealistic, and the Committee published findings recognizing a plurality of viewpoints (Bohleber et al., 2013, 2015). Similarly, Clinical Observation (CO) had an aim to enhance the study of session material by using dimensions drawn from validated methods (the PDM (2006) and the OPD (2008)), but this was integrated in psychoanalytic group work very similar to that of the Working Parties (Altmann de Litvan, 2014; Fitzpatrick-Hanly et al., 2021). Over time, CO has come to be considered as one of the Working Party-type endeavours, with activities in all three IPA regions (Chapter 10).

In 2015 a proposal was sent to the IPA Board to establish a new Committee within the IPA with a mandate to build bridges between the WPs and facilitate interregional communication. The IPA Working Parties Committee was formally set up in 2016 with members representing the different currents. The aim, while respecting the policies of the Regional Federations, was to collaborate with them to create an interregional scientific space for dialogue and scientific exchange among the WPs, thus broadening the scope of the IPA's scientific work and bringing the IPA and the Regional Federations closer together in joint scientific activities. As one means to this end, joint symposia between the IPA and the Regional Federations are held, both in the conferences of the Regional Federations and in IPA conferences, to share and discuss WP methods and findings. A related objective is to encourage the WPs to publish their findings in scientific papers aiming at a conceptual deepening of their reflections.

Working together in the Working Parties Committee and in the panels allowed the groups to get to know each other better and to move from what could sometimes be a climate of misunderstanding and mistrust to one of more active curiosity about the diverse orientations, reaching for a better understanding of commonalities and divergences. This book, on which work began in 2019, is one outcome of these efforts.

Reflections on the Scientific Status of Working Party Methods

From the outset, there have been questions about the scientific value of the Working Party effort. The "Ten Year European Scientific Initiative" explicitly announced the intention to improve our knowledge through systematic investigation. This led to debate about what can be considered "scientific" or not, what investigative methods are relevant for psychoanalysis, and whether systematic investigation is even possible in our field.

Science, in the broadest sense, involves curious and disciplined exploration. We are innately curious, asking: how do we solve this problem? Is there a better way to approach or to understand this? We pose questions and search for methods to explore them. The nature of the questions we ask determines our focus for exploration. So, too, does the cultural and scientific background in which we work. Sometimes our cultures, however, foreclose promising investigations: we need group membership, and groups may produce original work or instead may insist on conformity or on received doctrine. Some years ago, for example, Dr Suzanne Simard's ground-breaking research (2009) on hormonal exchanges between trees in a forest was disregarded because her findings were seen as inconsistent with existing theories.

Because of this ever-present possibility of bias, we must always address our explorations with lively but systematic approaches. It is crucial to consider our fields of interest with curiosity, depth, and relentlessness: what do we actually know that might help us understand this phenomenon? How do we know it? Is our evidence truly convincing? Psychoanalysts are faced with the same questions. Circular thinking is a constant risk, using language that is removed from actual data to spin explanations that will not hold up to close investigation. We tend to protect such explanations through *confirmation bias*, the tendency to prefer observations that fit with established views. As a result, we must keep pursuing our questions and testing our answers through multiple methods of inquiry.

Psychoanalysis is especially challenging for our investigative minds because it requires us to look carefully not only at the world, but also at ourselves. This is not only because we need to reflect on our minds and how we use them to understand or misunderstand what we see, which is a normal aspect of all enquiry. Nor is it just because our beliefs are linked to our position in our social and professional environment, a problem which psychoanalysis shares with all social sciences. Our special problem is that we can also become disturbed internally by the investigative process. Our explicit psychoanalytic theories can have multiple contact points with, and are often bolstered by, our implicit theories (Sandler, 1983). The latter can be grounded more in unconscious phantasy than in fact. Without realizing it, we can hold an explicit theory because it is important for our inner equilibrium, or we can think we are working on the basis of an explicit theory while actually we are influenced by a personal phantasy. Discovering this can be unsettling: the example of Dr A. is a case in point. The unconscious wish to avoid such alterations of our personal equilibrium can provide an additional source of bias. This is one of the reasons why the Working Party methods can be so helpful. Not only can colleagues from other psychoanalytic cultures help us to see our personal theoretical biases; their understanding presence can also be a precious source of support when we feel internally challenged.

To borrow a metaphor from Norman and Salomonsson (2005), doing research puts us back on the couch.

Comparisons With Other Research Methods

It is unscientific to believe pre-emptively that there is only one issue of clinical and theoretical import, or only one method to explore it. For example, considerable pressure has been placed on psychoanalysts to preferentially conduct randomized–controlled trials to demonstrate the various outcomes of psychoanalytic treatments. To focus exclusively on this important issue would be, however, to overlook other equally important questions and the multiple possibilities inherent in other or complementary methodologies, particularly qualitative ones.

Qualitative Research

Qualitative scientific methods rely on careful, systematic exploration, looking for potentially meaningful patterns. They are most often used to generate new observations and hypotheses, while quantitative research can test the hypotheses that are generated. Dr Simard, for example, first qualitatively observed that many different fungal species seemed to be interwoven into tree roots and began to systematically examine such interconnections microscopically. She then observed that the trees within a forest whose roots were interconnected via fungal networks seemed to be healthier than others. This led her to develop hypotheses about the tree-fungi-tree connections that she could later test quantitatively in her groundbreaking research.

For psychoanalytic research, qualitative investigations may include psychoanalytically structured interviews of subjects who share a similar condition: for example Blackburn et al.'s (2020) series of psychoanalytically informed interviews of chronic anorexic patients to better understand what, interpersonally and intra-psychically, contributed to the longevity of their symptoms. They may also be used to look closely at individual analytic sessions over time to consider which anchor points can be used to evaluate change and which interpretations seem to have led to shifts in an analytic process. Chapter 10 in this book from Clinical Observation provides a good illustration of such a project.

Some research projects combine both qualitative and quantitative modes of observation. Such mixed methods research led Marianne Leuzinger-Bohleber and her group, for example, to consider which psychoanalytic approaches worked best for a group of patients with chronic depression who had significant early trauma (2016). At the same time, she also quantitatively analyzed treatment outcomes for the entire depressive group.

Conceptual Research

Research in many fields is guided by conceptual analysis, which sometimes may precede, and at other times may follow up on, qualitative or quantitative research projects. Rachel Blass described conceptual research as the attempt to formally and systematically reason about working psychoanalytic hypotheses or about the methodologies behind some reported or planned research (summarized by Leuzinger-Bohleber, 2004; see also Leuzinger-Bohleber & Fischmann, 2006). Such reflections are intrinsically valuable: they may clarify what an investigation is designed to explore and how it is expected to do so. After a research project is completed, a conceptual assessment may be needed to re-examine the original assumptions in the light of the findings. Conceptual research has also led individual analysts or groups of analysts to rigorously investigate the methodology and concepts behind some accepted research reports.

In the Working Party on Psychosomatics, for example, analysts dissatisfied with current working concepts regarding what contributes to psychosomatic conditions engaged in a long-term project to explore multiple analyses of patients with such illnesses (see Chapter 9 in this book). As another example, one of the starting points for the study of first interviews by the EPF Working Party on Initiating Psychoanalysis was the failure of studies based on assessment of the patient's capacity for psychoanalysis to predict the outcome of the subsequent analyses. A new, psychoanalytically informed look at what happens in first interviews led this Working Party to conclude that the interviewing analyst and the patient work together to face a powerful unconscious "storm" that arises between them, rediscovering this concept from Bion (1979) as a potentially more useful explanatory model (Reith et al., 2018).

Action Research

The WP on Specificity was particularly interested in the transformational effect of psychoanalytic group work on all participants, including the presenting analyst and the investigative team. One of the ways they reflected on this was through the concept of "action research" developed by the social psychologist Kurt Lewin in 1944 as a methodology of research in the social sciences (Lewin, 1948; Marrow, 1969). In this model, doing research, taking action, and learning from action are combined and reinforce each other in simultaneous and recursive processes. As in qualitative research, hypothesis generation is part of the action research process, but the latter puts more accent on the transformative impact on the researchers and participants through their personal involvement.

This model can be compared to Freud's (1926) view that there is an "inseparable bond [or *"Junktim"* as he called it] between cure and research." For Freud, not only is the clinical work of the psychoanalyst a research activity, but moreover the curative effect of each psychoanalysis depends on the research that is done there. As a result, clinical work is the main way to gain psychoanalytic knowledge. Although in one sense the Working Parties can be thought of as doing a form of extra-clinical research, the fact that the workshops study psychoanalytic sessions and are transformed by their unconscious dynamics turns them into a clinical situation and thus into a form of clinical research. Because psychoanalytic research and the transformation of the participants (patients, clinicians, and researchers) go hand in hand, the scientific ideal of testing a clearly defined pre-established hypothesis can be inappropriate and can fail to capture significant processes.

Looking for Investigative Approaches
Specific to Psychoanalysis

In any field of study, the method must be adapted to the object and aim of the investigation. Dr Simard needed to begin with a microscope: a telescope or a high-energy particle collider would not have suited her purposes. The same is true for psychoanalysis: we need to find methods that capture the essentials of our field – our hypotheses about the working of the unconscious and about the unconscious transference and countertransference dynamics of the psychoanalytic session. How to do this is the source of legitimate concerns, creative explorations, and vibrant discussions about the most appropriate approaches, as noted earlier in the discussion about differences among Working Party approaches.

Thus, and as we have discussed, some Working Parties advocate using only investigative methodologies derived from the psychoanalytic method itself, such as group procedures based on evenly suspended attention and free association. This is often combined with attention to the group dynamics that can arise in the investigative groups, as possible expressions of the unconscious session dynamics not only in the minds of the analytic couple, but also in the minds of the analysts who explore the session reports. Such psychoanalytic work forms the backbone of all WP procedures that we know. The following vignette is an example of its power.

Dreaming the Countertransference

Dr B, in a different WP than Dr A, was impressed, while presenting his clinical material, by the workshop's ability to grasp aspects of his analytic relationship with the patient dating from a period after the sessions were reported and before their presentation. The sessions were from February and the material was presented in July. As the group reacted to the sessions presented, they began to have a countertransference reaction towards the patient's mother. "How did she allow the father to abuse the patient like that?" The presenting analyst was impacted silently, as within this WP's procedures, presenting analysts do not speak until specifically asked for their thoughts. However, he later revealed that this indignation with the mother had been precisely the prevalent feeling within the analytic duo during the period coming after the February sessions. The group had experienced the precise affective tone within this dyad although the analyst had not explicitly mentioned it. This form of unconscious communication, a method of knowledge specific to psychoanalysis, manifested itself in this example with all its force.

Dr B. came out of his first experience presenting clinical material in a WP with his faith in the psychoanalytic method strengthened. It was almost a lived rediscovery of the method. But more than that, the group's associative process and reverie produced a plethora of images that later resurfaced in Dr B.'s mind during his work with this patient, allowing them to access and understand new emotional experiences. It was as if the group had "dreamed" elements of the patient's and analyst's unconscious, helping the analyst to work with them later in the treatment.

Other Working Parties are interested to combine this psychoanalytic foundation with conceptual or qualitative research procedures. Each one has evolved a specific set of procedures that correspond to the questions they are addressing, the nature of their data and their guiding theoretical assumptions. The nature of the inquiry shapes the methodology. Their concern is then to ensure that their chosen approaches are compatible with psychoanalytic work. Doubts have been voiced about the relevance of qualitative methods to psychoanalysis and are legitimate if they amount to a shallow application of social science methods to our field. The WPs that use such methods, however, are usually careful to adapt them to the specificities of our domain and find that they enhance psychoanalytic exploration rather than impeding or distorting it.

As will be seen in the following chapters, all these approaches produce valuable results. This diversity of Working Party methods is in our view one of the most interesting and productive aspects of the whole endeavour. Many approaches need to be tried out to allow us to explore and compare their pertinence for psychoanalysis, and they may be found to be complementary. In our view the methodological debate cannot be decided theoretically. The final answer will be in cumulative experiences with, and in the outcomes of, these different ways of working.

Some Common Characteristics of Working Party Methods

It is possible, however, to discern core methods that most Working Parties seem to share. Regarding workshop procedures, each method specifies how long a workshop meets (from half a day to a day and a half) and the number of participants (typically 10 to 15). In general, each workshop begins with a presentation of clinical material from an analytic treatment (or, depending on the aims of the Working Party, from supervision or from first interviews prior to analysis). The presenter has been given specified instructions, for example about what kind of material to present, and whether or not to provide background and the patient's history. Each workshop has one or two moderators, and often an observer who keeps track of the proceedings and group processes.

The groups receive instructions about how to respond to the session material, either in a free associative style or with designated questions or frameworks in mind. The questions aim to focus on aspects of the material that the Working Party is studying and have often evolved and been refined over time. There may be several phases, for example asking the groups to begin with free-associative work and then to move on to the predefined questions or ones that have grown organically from the earlier phases. Working Parties do not use standardized scales, although in some instances they may borrow some ideas from them. The moderators have the task of facilitating a sense of safety in the group and promoting an open exchange of feelings, impressions, and ideas, as free as possible from theory or dogma. The intensity of the hours spent together increases group cohesion, augmented by a common set of questions and ways of reaching for answers.

The workshops are usually followed by further intensive study of the clinical material and workshop proceedings by a smaller investigative team. Frequently, these core teams have developed their own innovative ways of organizing or interrogating the data. In many Working Parties this analytic procedure is carried out in recursive steps, allowing the investigative team to take a second or third look at its own work.

These repetitive and numerous angles of observation mean that the initial object of study – the analyst/patient dyad – becomes triangulated in increasingly complex and expanded ways. The group of workshop participants who listen to the initial presentation constitutes a third-position platform from which to observe the initial dyad. Subsequently, the workshop frame shifts this third point of observation, so that the material is viewed from different angles. The group may be asked to try to examine itself and the group processes so that another observation point is constructed. When the investigative team later examines the clinical material and processes that were presented in the initial dyad and then arose in the workshop's response, the workshop group becomes the object of study from yet another perspective. Thus, the Working Party methods are constructed upon the common theoretical and technical conviction of the importance of triangulation, in the sense of finding ways to stand outside the self, the therapeutic dyad, or a professional group, to observe and study what is going on in the psychoanalytic situation. This expresses shared common values of self-reflection and the need for finding more and more refined ways of reflecting together on the psychoanalytic process in systematic and relevant ways.

This ever-expanding set of triangulations, reflections, and decentering begins with the initial presentation: as the Working Party on Listening to Listening puts it: "There is often a moment when the presenter becomes curious about his/her own presentation, and decenters his/her own listening" (see Chapter 6). The same triangulating process has extended to the larger analytic/scientific community as the Working Parties describe their methods and findings in conferences, publications, and now in this book.

The practical data collection and analysis substantiating such work starts with the written session transcripts brought by the presenting analyst. All the workshop proceedings, including the initial presentation and the participants' responses to it, are recorded in some manner. In most cases the workshops are audio recorded for later reference. The recordings can be transcribed, or more usually the workshop observer takes scrupulous notes and transcribes them, referring back to the audio recordings for specific sequences. These transcriptions are then used by the smaller investigative groups for the next steps of data analysis.

When the investigative teams revisit this workshop material, it is usually both with free-associative work and with certain specific or open-ended questions in mind. Significant recurring patterns of sequences are noted. Unusual one-time phenomena are also noted. In the Comparative Clinical Methods Working Party, for instance, it was noted that analysts do not always work in predictable conscious ways: an analyst who believes s/he works consistently within the transference, in fact works in a different manner, more focused on empathic mirroring (Rudden & Bronstein, 2015; Chapter 4). In the chapters that follow each working party will give examples of the kind of data that they have found, the type of analyses done, and any conclusions drawn from them. Conclusions are drawn slowly, tentatively, when patterns accumulate over many instances and across levels of analysis. When no more new hypotheses, ideas, or meanings arise from a piece of clinical material, after multiple eyes and ears have been exposed to it, it may be considered "saturated." The utilization of standard procedures in repetitive meetings of each working party means that hypotheses can be "tested" through multiple comparisons of the clinical phenomena that emerge.

All Working Parties have described how groups can find themselves enacting aspects of the unconscious dynamics embedded in the sessions under study. Such events can be highly informative if, at some stage, and with the support of their methods, the workshop or investigative team can recognize them and elaborate on their unconscious meaning. Thus, the specific methodology that each Working Party has developed can be thought of as analogous to the psychoanalytic frame and is usually explicitly or implicitly understood as such. Currently psychoanalysts conceptualize the frame not as static or concrete, but fluid and elastic, co-created and contextual, less as a noun than as a verb: "to frame," or "framing" (Bass, 2007; Gonzalez, 2020; Levine, 2009). For the Working Parties "to frame" takes on the meaning "to create a system or a method" and also "to enclose or contain." In this latter sense, many of the Working Parties conceptualize their group processes in Bion's terms (1962) as a container for the strong, often unmetabolized affects and unconscious phantasies that arise as they work with the presented material. Chapters 3 and 5 on Specificity and Initiating Psychoanalysis are examples. In yet another sense, the Working Parties use the concept of frame as a triangulation procedure to highlight or to focus on one element of a complex matrix to study it closely, as illustrated by many approaches in this book. Finally, the method as frame may itself become a focus of study when group participants try to deviate from the procedures or respond to chance disruptions of the setting in which they work.

Validity

Psychoanalysts have hotly debated the relative benefits of the different major approaches to securing knowledge in the field:

- Observing phenomena in their consulting room (Freud's "*Junktim*");

- Comparing cases qualitatively and allowing patterns to emerge from many cases (qualitative methods);
- Or actively testing existing hypotheses, usually with standardized methods (quantitative research).

This discussion involves questions about the validity of each approach, i.e., whether it applies adequate methods ensuring that its findings are meaningful and trustworthy. There are specific definitions of validity in empirical science (Cook & Beckman, 2006) as well as in qualitative research (Creswell, 2014). Validity in empirical science includes several aspects, in particular: *convergent validity* (new approaches essentially converge in important ways with what is already acknowledged as valid in the field); *construct validity* (a measure is internally consistent in its construction and the study as a whole is consistent in its questions and methodology); and *predictive validity* (what is claimed can actually predict results in a study and in future ones).

Qualitative researchers within the social sciences and currently within psychoanalysis have developed complementary procedures for determining the reliability and validity of many differently derived findings. These have proven very useful for psychoanalysts engaged in qualitative research projects (for a clinical example, see Tillman et al., 2011, 2017; for an overview of psychoanalytic qualitative research in psychoanalysis, see Wallerstein, 2009; and for a general overview of methods for establishing the interpretive validity of qualitative findings, see Denzin & Lincoln, 1998).

We must adapt this extremely important issue to our field and suggest, as a first step in this direction, that in its most general sense validity means:

- Research questions make sense in the context of what is known about the field and are in principle answerable using appropriate methods.
- The chosen methods are constantly reexamined to assess whether they really address those questions and how.
- They are applied reliably, meaning that they can be used in the same way by different researchers and that there is a consistency of their findings over studies and especially within a given study.
- The findings are examined for possible alternative explanations.
- Transparency, allowing independent evaluation of the reported findings against the data provided, is an important aspect.

The purpose of concerns with both validity and reliability is to ensure that data are sound and replicable and that their results are accurate and useful. Such judgements will of course depend on thorough familiarity with the field of study, as well as on confrontation with multiple viewpoints, including from outside the field, to safeguard against circular reasoning and ensure that alternative explanations are not neglected.

There are special challenges and opportunities here for psychoanalysis. Because of the profoundly personal nature of psychoanalytic practice (each patient-analyst pair will have both universal and totally individual characteristics) and research (each analyst or group will respond in both common and unique ways to session material submitted for examination), reproducibility in psychoanalytic research will not take the form of an exact replication of identical or nearly phenomena, but rather of recognizable, recurring dynamic patterns underlying the infinite variety of phenomena (Reith et al., 2018). Moreover, given the highly specialized epistemic foundations of psychoanalysis (evenly suspended attention, receptiveness, openness to transformation and self-reflective functioning of the analyst, usually in the encounter of two or more minds), one aspect of pattern recognition in our profession will necessarily be based on intersubjective consensus by experienced psychoanalysts who recognize each other's assessment of a clinical sequence, or of comparable sequences in plural cases. Such intersubjective consensus concerns not only phenomena but also their meaning, and involves multiple perspectives and correspondences not only between observation and theory but also between different intra-subjective experiences, between conscious and preconscious, and between reason and affect (Civitarese, 2018). Much of this takes place unconsciously and can only be understood *après coup*.

This intersubjective validation is the object of further debate between those who find it in

- A common search for recurring dynamic patterns or for particularly interesting observed phenomena within an accumulated series of case studies, or in
- A growing spiral of individual associations to each case, leading to a progressive expansion and enrichment of meaning.

Many would probably think that these aspects are complementary, since an unlimited expansion of meaning could ultimately result in meaningless dispersion without a recognition of patterns, and vice versa, patterns would be sterile if they did not give birth to new meaning.

- In addition, and knowing the self-reflective nature of psycho-analytic work, observing how groups of analysts respond to the material they are studying, and the kinds of group phenomena that emerge (agreements, conflicts, unnoticed divisions, enact-ments, or regressions), will be another important component of uniquely psychoanalytic methods for data analysis and control-ling for bias.

All the preceding are part of what makes psychoanalytic work lively and convincing. Part of the impetus behind the Working Party endeavour, however, arises from the hope that such psycho-analytic sources of insight can be augmented and refined by using additional systematic procedures. In this view, the critical, third-person, or triangulating perspective offered by such methods does not only help to ensure reliability and validity; it also empowers psychoanalytic understanding (Bernardi, 2017; Glover & Reith, 2021).

In their chapters for this book, many Working Parties offer examples of the clinical sessions presented to their groups, as well as the findings suggested by the analysts who listened and reflected upon this clinical material. These data and the conclusions reached by the Working Parties offer a unique opportunity for readers to form an independent opinion of the validity and reliability of both their methods and the conclusions offered. Over time, the Working Parties may of course need to further explore and define their criteria to determine the validity and reliability of their con-clusions and expose them to the scrutiny of their psychoanalytic and non-psychoanalytic colleagues. Meanwhile the strength of the Working Parties is that they examine a variety of hypotheses about how psychoanalysis works and how psychoanalysts understand their encounter with their analysands. The fact that multiple psycho-analysts consider the presented material at multiple levels of the Working Party process and come to a consensus on their observa-tions ensures the reliability of the findings by most standards, while the plurality of perspectives provides an overall safeguard against circular or rule-bound reasoning.

Structure of the Book

The different Working Parties and similar endeavours are illustrated in Chapters 2 to 10. We have asked each group to present their history, aims, and methods, and give an example of their findings. Each chapter is self-contained; readers may want to read them in order, or dip into them according to their inclination. They will find that chapters are strikingly individual in style and content and that the accent chosen by the authors ranges from a reflection on methods adequate for psychoanalytic research to illustrative findings, and to the relevance of both methods and findings for psychoanalytic training and clinical practice. Although each chapter was discussed at length in our Committee and with the authors to improve their presentation and clarity, we did not want to strive for uniformity and decided to respect the authors' ultimate choices as an expression of the richness of the field. In this first introductory chapter, elaborated by our Committee, we have tried to highlight some of the points of convergence among the different Working Parties; but now space must be left for the divergences. We thank the authors for having understood this working spirit and for the quality and originality of their contributions. All necessary measures have been taken by the authors and their collaborators to ensure that the confidentiality of the clinical cases illustrating the chapters has been respected.

The book ends with an erudite and thoughtful assessment by Patrizia Giampieri-Deutsch examining the contributions of the Working Parties to psychoanalysis and psychoanalytic research, in Chapter 11. We are extremely grateful for her marvellous work of synthesizing this burgeoning field.

The book the reader has in their hands is, in its achievements and its imperfections, a product of an eventful history and a demonstration of ongoing developments. We consider it as an exploratory and open initiative, an introduction to the potential of the Working Party movement and by no means as a "definitive" statement. Clearly much more work will be needed, but we will have achieved our aims if this book provides some impetus in that direction.

Note

1 By the members of the Working Parties Committee of the International Psychoanalytical Association who have edited this book: Ruggero Levy, Chair; Bernard Reith, Co-chair for Europe; Marie G. Rudden,

Co-chair for North America; Agustina Fernández, Co-chair for Latin America; Nancy Kulish, Member for North America; Leopoldo Bleger, Member for Europe; and Inés Bayona Villegas, Member for Latin America.

Bibliography

Altmann de Litvan, M. (Ed.) (2014). *Time for change: Tracking transformations in psychoanalysis – The Three-Level Model.* Karnac.

Anzieu, D. (1999). *Le Groupe et l'Inconscient: L'imaginaire groupal.* 3rd edition. Dunod.

Balint, M. (1964). *The doctor, his patient and the illness.* Pitman Medical Publishing.

Bass, A. (2007). When the frame doesn't fit the picture. *Psychoanal: Dialogues, 17,* 1–27.

Bernardi, R. (1989). The role of paradigmatic determinants in psychoanalytic understanding. *International Journal of Psychoanalysis, 70,* 341–357.

Bernardi, R. (1992). On pluralism in psychoanalysis. *Psychoanalytic Inquiry, 12,* 506–525.

Bernardi, R. (2002). The need for true controversies in psychoanalysis. *International Journal of Psychoanalysis, 83,* 851–873.

Bernardi, R. (2017). A common ground in clinical discussion groups: Intersubjective resonance and implicit operational theories. *International Journal of Psycho-Analysis, 98,* 1291–1309.

Bion, W. R. (1962). *Learning from experience.* Karnac.

Bion, W. R. (1987). Making the best of a bad job. In W. R. Bion, & F. Bion (Eds.), *Clinical seminars and four papers* (pp. 247–257). Fleetwood Press. (Original work published 1979).

Blackburn, B., O'Connor, J., & Parsons, H. (2020). Becoming needless: A psychoanalytically informed qualitative study exploring the interpersonal and intrapsychic experiences of longstanding anorexia nervosa. *International Journal of Applied Psychoanalytic Studies,* 03.11.2020: doi.org/10.1002/APS.1679

Boesky, D. (2008). *Psychoanalytic disagreements in context.* Rowman & Littlefield.

Bohleber, W., Fonagy, P., Jiménez, J. P., Scarfone, D., Varvin, S., & Zysman, S. (2013). Towards a better use of psychoanalytic concepts: A model illustrated using the concept of enactment. *International Journal of Psychoanalysis, 94,* 501–530.

Bohleber, W., Jiménez, J. P., Scarfone, D., Varvin, S., & Zysman, S. (2015). Unconscious phantasy and its conceptualizations: An attempt at conceptual integration. *International Journal of Psychoanalysis, 96,* 705–730.

Bryant, A., & Charmaz, K. (2007). Grounded theory in historical perspective: An epistemological account. In A. Bryant, & K. Charmaz (Eds.), *The Sage handbook of grounded theory* (pp. 31–57). Sage.

Canestri, J. (2008). *Psychoanalysis: From practice to theory*. Whurr.

Canestri, J. (2012). *Putting theories to work: How are theories actually used in practice?* Karnac.

Charmaz, K. (2006). *Constructing grounded theory: A practical guide through qualitative analysis*. Sage.

Charmaz, K., & Bryant, A. (2011). Grounded theory and credibility. In D. Silverman (Ed.), *Qualitative research: Issues of theory, methods, and practice*. 3rd edition, (pp. 291–309). Sage.

Civitarese, G. (2018). Truth as immediacy and unison: A new common ground in psychoanalysis? Commentary on essays addressing "Is truth relevant?" In *Sublime subjects – Aesthetic experience and intersubjectivity in psychoanalysis* (Chapter 8, pp. 121–156). Routledge.

Cook, D. A., & Beckman, T. J. (2006). Current concepts in validity and reliability for psychometric instruments: Theory and application. *American Journal of Medicine, 119* (2), 166, e7–e16.

Creswell, R. (2014). *Research design: Qualitative, quantitative and mixed methods approaches*. Sage.

Denzin, N. K., & Lincoln, Y. S. (1998). *Collecting and interpreting qualitative materials*. Sage.

Donnet, J. L. (2005). *La situation analysante*. Presses Universitaires de France.

Ehrlich, L. T., Kulish, N. M., Hanley, M. A., Robinson, M., & Rothstein, A. (2017). Supervisory countertransferences and impingements in evaluating readiness for graduation: Always present, routinely under-recognized. *International Journal of Psychoanalysis, 98*, 491–516.

Erlich-Ginor, M. (2010). The EPF working party on education – An overview. *European Psychoanalytical Federation Bulletin, 64* (Supplement), 33–56.

Faimberg, H. (2005). *The telescoping of generations: Listening to the narcissistic links between generations*. Routledge.

Faimberg, H. (2019). Basic theoretical assumptions underpinning Faimberg's method: "Listening to listening". *International Journal of Psychoanalysis, 100*, 447–462.

Fitzpatrick-Hanly, M. A., Altmann, M., & Bernardi, R. (Eds.) (2021). *Change through time in psychoanalysis: Transformations and interventions: The Three-Level Model*. Routledge.

Forrester, J. (2017). *Thinking in cases*. Polity Press.

Freud, S. (1925). An autobiographical study. In J. Strachey (Ed. & Trans.), *The standard edition of the complete psychological works of Sigmund Freud* (Vol. 20, pp. 1–74). Hogarth Press, 1959.

Freud, S. (1926). The question of lay analysis. In J. Strachey (Ed. & Trans.), *The standard edition of the complete psychological works of Sigmund Freud* (Vol. 20, pp. 177–258). Hogarth Press, 1959.

Frisch, S., Bleger, L., & Séchaud, E. (2010). The specificity of psychoanalytic treatment today (WPSPTT). *Psychoanalysis in Europe: Bulletin of the European psychoanalytical federation, 64* (Supplement), 81–110.

Geverif, R. (2017a). Dialogic and dialectic: Clarifying an important distinction. www.rupertwegerif.name/blog/dialogic-and-dialectic-clarifying-an-important-distinction, 29.06.2017, accessed 04.12.2021.

Geverif, R. (2017b). Dialogic space and why we need it. www.rupertwegerif.name/blog/dialogic-space-why-we-need-it, 05.09.2017, accessed 04.12.2021.

Glaser, B., & Strauss, A. L. (1967). *The discovery of grounded theory: Strategies for qualitative research*. Aldine de Gruyter.

Glover, W., & Reith, B. (2021). Working parties as clinical research. In M. Altmann de Litvan (Ed.), *Clinical research in psychoanalysis: Theoretical basis and experiences through Working Parties* (pp. 151–160). Routledge.

Gonzalez, F. J. (2020). First world problems and gated communities of the mind: An ethics of place in psychoanalysis. *Psychoanalytic Quarterly, 89,* 741–770.

Green, A. (2005). The illusion of common ground and mythical pluralism. *International Journal of Psychoanalysis, 86,* 627–632.

Habermas, J. (1984). *The theory of communicative action* (Vol. 1), T. McCarthy (Trans.). Polity Press.

Hinze, E. (2015). What do we learn in psychoanalytic training? *International Journal of Psychoanalysis, 96* (3), 755–771.

Kaës, R. (2005). *La parole et le lien: Processus associatifs et travail psychique dans les groupes*. 2nd édition. Dunod.

Leuzinger-Bohleber, M. (2004). What does conceptual research have to offer? *International Journal of Psychoanalysis, 85,* 1477–1478.

Leuzinger-Bohleber, M., & Fischmann, T. (2006). What is conceptual research in psychoanalysis? *International Journal of Psychoanalysis, 87,* 1355–1386.

Leuzinger-Bohleber, M., Stuhr, U., Ruger, B., & Beutel, M. (2016). Pluralistic approaches to the study of process and outcome in psychoanalysis: The LAC depression study: Case in point. *Psychoanalytic Psychotherapy, 30,* 4–22.

Levine, A. (2009). Bending the frame and judgment calls in everyday practice. *Journal of the American Psychoanalytic Association, 57,* 1209–1213.

Lewin, K. (1948) Action research and minority problems. In G. W. Lewin (Ed.), *Resolving social conflicts*. Harper & Row.

Loch, W. (1995). *Theorie und Praxis von Balint-Gruppen*. Edition Discord.

Marrow, A. J. (1969). *The practical theorist: The life and work of Kurt Lewin.* Basic Books.

Morin, E. (1982). *Science avec conscience.* Seuil.

Morin, E. (2005). *Introduction à la pensée complexe.* Seuil.

Moss, D. (2018). On a regressive feature of applied psychoanalysis. In *At war with the obvious: Disruptive thinking in psychoanalysis* (pp. 77–89). Routledge.

Nikulin, D. (2010). *Dialectic and dialogue.* Stanford University Press.

Norman, J., & Salomonsson, B. (2005). "Weaving thoughts": A method for presenting and commenting psychoanalytic case material in a peer group. *International Journal of Psychoanalysis, 86,* 1281–1298.

OPD Task Force (2008). *Operationalized psychodynamic diagnosis manual of diagnosis and treatment planning.* Hogrefe and Huber.

PDM. (2006). *Psychodynamic diagnostic manual.* Alliance of Psychoanalytic Organizations.

Reith, B., Lagerlöf, S., Crick, P., Møller, M., & Skale, E. (Eds.) (2012). *Initiating psychoanalysis: Perspectives.* Routledge.

Reith, B., Møller, M., Boots, J., Crick, P., Gibeault, A., Jaffè, R., Lagerlöf, S., & Vermote, R. (2018). *Beginning analysis: On the processes of initiating psychoanalysis.* Routledge.

Rudden, M., & Bronstein, A. (2015). Transference, the relationship and the analyst as object: Findings from the North American Comparative Clinical Methods Working Party. *International Journal of Psychoanalysis, 96,* 681–703.

Salomonsson, B. (2012). Psychoanalytic case presentations in a weaving thoughts group: On countertransference and group dynamics. *International Journal of Psychoanalysis, 93,* 917–937.

Sandler, J. (1983). Reflections on some relations between psychoanalytic concepts and psychoanalytic practice. *International Journal of Psychoanalysis, 64,* 35–45.

Schülein, J. A. (2003). On the logic of psychoanalytic theory. *International Journal of Psychoanalysis, 84,* 315–330.

Simard, S. W. (2009). The foundational role of mycorrhizal networks in self-organization of interior douglas-fir forests. *Forest Ecology and Management, 258,* S95–S107.

Tillman, J., Clemence, A. J., & Stevens, J. (2011). Mixed methods research design for pragmatic psychoanalytic studies. *Journal of the American Psychoanalytic Association, 59,* 1027–1040.

Tillman, J., et al. (2017). The persistent shadow of suicide ideation and attempts in a high-risk group of psychiatric patients: A focus for intervention. *Comprehensive Psychiatry, 77,* 20–26.

Tuckett, D. (1994). Developing a grounded hypothesis to understand a clinical process: The role of conceptualisation in validation. *International Journal of Psychoanalysis, 75,* 1159–1180.

Tuckett, D. (2000). The EPF policy and objectives for the next four years. *European Psychoanalytical Federation Bulletin, 54,* 111–118.

Tuckett, D. (2002). Presidential address: The new style conference and developing a peer culture in European psychoanalysis. *European Psychoanalytical Federation Bulletin, 56,* 32–46.

Tuckett, D. (2003). Presidential address: A Ten Year European Scientific Initiative. *European Psychoanalytical Federation Bulletin, 57,* 7–22.

Tuckett, D. (2004). Presidential address: Building a psychoanalysis based on confidence in what we do. *European Psychoanalytical Federation Bulletin, 58,* 5–20.

Tuckett, D. (2005). Does anything go? *International Journal of Psychoanalysis, 86,* 31–49.

Tuckett, D., Basile, R., Birksted-Breen, D., Böhm, T., Denis, P., Ferro, A., Hinz, H., Jemstedt, A., Mariotti, P., & Schubert, J. (2008). *Psychoanalysis comparable and incomparable: The evolution of a method to describe and compare psychoanalytic approaches.* Routledge.

Wallerstein, R. S. (1988). One psychoanalysis or many? *International Journal of Psychoanalysis, 69,* 5–21.

Wallerstein, R. S. (1990). Psychoanalysis: The common ground. *International Journal of Psychoanalysis, 71,* 3–20.

Wallerstein, R. S. (2009). What kind of research in psychoanalytic science? *International Journal of Psychoanalysis, 90,* 109–133.

Wiener-Margulies, M. (2014). Out of the box and into the Working Parties: A journey well worth the risk. *The Candidate Connection: Newsletter of the APsaA Candidates' Council, 16,* 3–5.

2

END OF TRAINING PROJECT/MIND OF THE SUPERVISOR

Situations With Institutional Impingement

Eike Hinze, Nancy Kulish and Marianne Robinson

Historical Background and Development of the End of Training Project (ETEP)

The Working Party on Education (WPE)

The End of Training/Mind of the Supervisor Working Party is a descendent of the Working Party on Education (WPE). In her overview on the WPE 2009, Mira Erlich-Ginor (2010) clearly describes the challenging task of this working party: "How is it possible to explore psychoanalytic education that involves candidates, training analysts, teachers, has different stages – admission, transmission, qualification, to mention just a few of the components that make up what we mean by a 'system of psychoanalytic education'" (p. 1–2). Recognizing that no one single research project could adequately address the variety of issues that comprise psychoanalytic education, a series of six studies with different methodologies appropriate to different aspects of this complex field were created. Different members of the WPE collaborated in each while the whole group served as a container in which these projects were discussed. Mary Target (2001), the first chair of the WPE, laid the foundation for each of these studies by collecting the existing

DOI: 10.4324/9781032656311-2

literature on psychoanalytic training. The six individual studies addressed the following issues:

1. Who does what? (the mapping of factual aspects of training)
2. The spectrum of views on psychoanalytic training in Europe
3. Becoming and being a training analyst
4. Studying the effectiveness of the End of Training Evaluation
5. Determining psychoanalytic competency
6. Studying the ending process of personal analysis

A description of these projects can be found in Mira Erlich-Ginor's overview (2009). Whereas all of these projects came to an eventual end, the End of Training Evaluation Project (ETEP) flourished and became the successor of the WPE in 2010. The chairs of WPE were Mary Target, Gabriele Junkers, and Mira Erlich-Ginor.

The End of Training Evaluation Project (ETEP)

Under the umbrella of the European Psychoanalytic Federation, ETEP was active from 2010 to 2014, chaired by Eike Hinze (2014) then was followed by the Working Party on Exploring Training Process and Practice (ETPP), which is still working. During the four years it existed, ETEP contributed to psychoanalytic education in meaningful ways, attracting numerous training analysts to its workshops that took place at the annual EPF Forums on Training, EPF Conferences, and International IPA Congresses. ETEP methodology, described in detail in the second part of this chapter, continues to be utilized by groups in North and Latin America.

The paper by David Tuckett (2005) "Does anything go?: Towards a framework for the more transparent assessment of psychoanalytic competence" can be regarded as a founding stone of ETEP. Three core papers have been published thus far describing the developmental process in the project and its initial scientific results. Junkers et al. (2008) reported the initial findings of the discussions at the EPF Working Party about how supervising analysts think about evaluation and what concepts and categories they use when they evaluate psychoanalytic competence at the end of training. This enterprise was met with much interest and open-mindedness.

In 2015, Eike Hinze summarized more than a decade of work by the EPF Working Party End of Training Evaluation Project (ETEP) on agreed-upon requirements for a successful ending of psychoanalytic training. Analysts of many theoretical orientations could agree on the following criteria: the ability to understand the emotional demand of a patient in every session, to appreciate the value of free association, to preserve a neutral stance, to think in terms of transference and countertransference, and to think conceptually about what is happening and what one is doing in *the session*.

The emerging findings from the ETEP indicated that analysts were anxious about evaluation and making definite decisions about candidates, and about exposing their work as supervisors. Based on experiences in the ETEP and other settings, Shmuel Erlich and Mira Erlich-Ginor (2018) explored the "nearly universal difficulty surrounding the evaluation of progress and competence of candidates in psychanalytic training" (p. 1131). They found vast institutional differences of opinion about the place of evaluation and the nature of its implementation, and cited examples of "supervisory anxiety" reflecting the ambiguity surrounding the role and authority of the supervisor. Erlich and Erlich-Ginor suggested that in this area psychoanalytic institutes tend to operate under Bion's basic assumptions of group functioning: fight-flight, dependency, and pairing. Although the ETEP now does not work as an officially acknowledged and financially supported EPF Working Party, it continues in North and South America, has spread to the worldwide psychoanalytic community, and has become a cornerstone in discussing psychoanalytic training.

Format of the Working Party

The format of the ETEP group discussion is designed to help get inside the mind of the supervisor as he or she supervises and evaluates candidates for readiness to graduate. In a two-day workshop, a specially trained moderator meets with a group of eight to twelve supervising analysts from different IPA institutes. A supervising analyst presents prepared verbatim material from supervisions of one or two psychoanalytic candidates. The presenter supplies background on the patient and supervisee, as well as information about the training program in his or her institute. The group is provided with material in advance about the purposes and format of the Working Party.

The presenting supervisor provides detailed process notes from the analytic sessions that the candidate reports and detailed descriptions of what was said and occurred in actual supervisory sessions. At the beginning of the meeting, the group is instructed to focus on the supervisory process and the mind of the supervisor, and not on the dynamics or techniques of treating the case. The moderators intervene when necessary to keep the group focused on the supervisor's mind. Presentation of each case is usually allotted at least three hours. A reporter takes detailed notes of the proceedings. It is the group's task to try to understand and to articulate what the explicit and implicit criteria the supervisor is using to evaluate the candidate – what he or she has in mind as necessary capacities for a graduate analyst, and the criteria about what constitutes individual pathology and analytic process. The presenter is asked not to discuss the criteria he or she uses in evaluating psychoanalytic progress until the group has expressed its observations and speculations about this. Many of the findings evolve directly and immediately from group discussions in the Working Party. This focus on understanding what is going on in the supervisor's mind helps to lessen possible effects arising from participants' individual theories or biases. Typically, three additional hours are devoted to a discussion of the particular institutional pressures and parameters relevant for the supervisor as well, and a comparison among the group participants of the institutional policies and issues in their particular institutes.

After the meetings, the two moderators discuss their impressions and ideas about the workshop and the material with each other. The reports are sent to all participants and to the presenters for corrections and additions. Later, the core members of the Working Party meet to go over, in detail, the available supervisory material and group responses taken from reports of the Working Party group discussions. In these special meetings, reports of different Working Parties are reread and compared to explore general themes or phenomena that may be discerned about the supervisory situation.

Through this process, the Working Party has been able to garner a strikingly common set of criteria to access candidates' readiness to progress and to graduate used by analysts around the world, such as the ability to contain affect, set boundaries, deal with transference, make use of countertransference, etc. These results are described in a series of papers (Junkers et al., 2005; Hinze, 2013) and have been utilized by progression committees in various institutes to clarify criteria for graduation.

Moreover, with this approach, the Working Party on ETEP has been able to elucidate psychic processes that go on in the mind of supervisors during supervision. In addition to trying to understand the supervisor's explicit and implicit assumptions about analysis and readiness for graduation in a candidate – and what criteria he or she uses to make these assessments, the group also found patterns and signs that may help to elucidate blind spots, transferences, counter-transferences, and other unconscious processes in the supervisor. In this process, participants pay attention to what feelings arise in the group process while listening both to the case and to the supervision. The moderator facilitates a group discussion that can lead to conclusions about common criteria for graduation, and to clarification about what factors might interfere with or facilitate the supervisory process, especially with respect to evaluation of candidate progress.

Unconscious Processes in Supervisors' Minds

While there are abundant writings on supervision, including supervisory countertransference (Caligor, 1981; Strean, 1991; Lester & Robertson, 1995; Skolnikoff, 1997; Berman, 2000; Jacobs, 2001; Weinstein et al., 2009), there are relatively few papers containing detailed examples of supervisory countertransference from supervisory sessions. Furthermore, little has been written in depth about supervisory countertransferences and other unconscious reactions that relate specifically to supervisors' function as evaluators of candidate progression, despite this being one of the most important functions of supervisors in psychoanalytic institutions.

Using detailed qualitative data from in-depth reports of supervisory hours, we have demonstrated that in their function as evaluators, supervisors are subject to internal and external pressures in various combinations which, if not recognized, may in turn create countertransferential blind spots and make them more prone to enactments. We found that supervisory countertransferences (and their manifestation in parallel enactments) are often under-recognized and under-utilized, and their impact on supervisors' ability to evaluate candidates' progress toward graduation is underappreciated.

39

Theoretical Background:
Countertransference in Supervision

The first discussions of the unconscious enactments within the supervisory situation appear in the literature on the "parallel process." Searles (1955), Ekstein and Wallerstein (1958), and Arlow (1963) describe the striking phenomena of the supervisee unconsciously replicating with his supervisor aspects of how the patient behaved toward or experienced him or her. These papers, written from the vantage point of a one-person analytic perspective, emphasize the supervisee's identification with the patient and the need to share unconscious content with the supervisor.

Soon, however, the discussion widened. In a comprehensive research project that examines data from supervisors and students in an outpatient clinic, Doehrman (1976) describes being struck both by the recurring parallel process and *the complexity of the supervisory relationship.* Supervisors, too, become embroiled in transference and countertransference binds in supervision that replicate the binds found in the treatment. Unlike the original formulations of parallel process as a one-way process beginning with the patient, this study found that the supervisor may generate anxiety in the therapist, which is then acted out by the therapist with his or her patient. Furthermore, the supervisor could not see these binds clearly until they were discussed with a third party. Gediman and Wolkenfeld (1980) also point out that in the parallel process there can be a reverse influence in which the analyst/patient dyad reenacts events from the supervisory situation.

Teitelbaum (1990) has coined the term *supertransference* to refer to the supervisor's unconscious contributions to the supervision. He underscores the strong influence of "such factors as the supervisor's narcissistic investment and needs, his or her expectations of the therapist, reactions to the personality of the therapist, and counterreactions to the therapist's transferences to the supervisor" on supervisees' capacity to participate effectively and use the supervision (p. 256).

Once analysts began to appreciate the complexity of the supervisory relationship and the fact of the supervisor's transferences, they then confront a substantive question as to whether the notion of a parallel process continues to be helpful. Observing that detailed examples of supervisory countertransferences were not present in the literature, Stimmel (1995) cautions that the use of the parallel process phenomena can serve as a resistance to the awareness of the supervisor's countertransferences and become "good places to hide unwanted transferences" (p. 615). Other writers (Baudry, 1993; Miller & Twomey, 1999; Werbart, 2007) have outlined the limitations of the concept of parallel process and criticized it as too vague or reductionistic and therefore of restricted or no clinical value.

On the other hand, Mendelsohn (2012) suggests that parallel enactment is a powerful explanatory concept when seen as the result of the process of projective identification. Mendelsohn views parallel process as a "kind of countertransference" (p. 311) initiated by the patient's (and at times the candidate's or the supervisor's) projective identifications. Bion's ideas (1965) about the communicative aspects of projective identification are relevant in this regard. He developed the concept of container/contained as an interpersonal exchange in which the presence of not-yet-metabolized sensations and experience (the contained) are unconsciously expressed for the purpose of being received and metabolized in a receptive relationship (container) which, using metabolizing capacities (alpha-function), returns the experience in ways that consider the "sender's" readiness and ability to receive and make use of it for the purpose of growing. This model seems naturally applicable, not only to the supervising situation but also to the End of Training/Mind of the Supervisor Working Party group whose function then can be seen as a potential containing and metabolizing entity for the supervisory couple that is being presented.

Findings: Supervisory Transferences/ Countertransferences

We have found that the supervisor is subject to multiple, diverse, and, at times, ongoing internal and external impingements on his or her ability to evaluate the candidate's progress. As the Working Party groups tried to identify the criteria used by supervisors in their assessments of analytic competency, they also began to notice silent forces at play in the supervisors' minds. *It was a surprising finding that in all the cases that we examined, such unconscious and preconscious impingements were always at play – sometimes facilitating, sometimes interfering, sometimes both.* In every case, the Working Party group was able to

41

observe such unconscious reactions, including noticeable counter-transferences and blind–spots, in every supervisory pair and in every supervisor, whether or not he or she was senior and experienced and regardless of theoretical orientation. These internal processes include transferences to the person of the candidate or patient, countertrans-ferences to the patient's and candidate's transferences, unconscious identifications and projections which reverberated among the three parties, and a myriad of other internal psychic phenomena, such as narcissistic issues, conflicts, anxieties, etc.

These results are detailed and discussed in an article published in *IJP* (Ehrlich et al., 2017). These findings fall into two categories: those arising within the supervisory triad, such as the countertrans-ference reactions mentioned earlier, and those arising from institu-tional influences (while at the same time recognizing that in reality these categories often overlap).

In this chapter we focus on two aspects of this complex supervi-sory situation: first, how silent institutional influences operate on the supervisor, and second, how these external pressures may interact with unconscious internal states in the supervisor's mind and rever-berate in the supervisory situation. Brief case examples are provided from specific supervisory situations.

Institutional Impingements, Including the Imperative to Evaluate

There are wide differences in the cultures, policies, and procedures of psychoanalytic training programs across the world which provide the silent but influential context for the supervisory process and the evaluation of candidate progression (Jaffe, 2001; Zaslavsky et al., 2005; Ehrlich et al., 2017). These institutional factors which oper-ate silently and unnoticed are often unknown, unappreciated, and unconscious, taken for granted as the air we breathe. These variables affect the supervisory and analytic dyads in basic ways – setting the frames of their work. They seep into the minds of the three parties, both consciously and unconsciously, and are internalized.

The composition of the Working Parties with participants from around the world has afforded the opportunity to examine and compare the differing institutional effects on the supervisory process depend-ing upon the particular psychoanalytic training program in which the supervisor and candidate work. Based on her work with ETE Working

Party groups, Mira Erlich-Ginor from Israel has articulated seven core areas in which psychoanalytic training institutes differ. These concern requirements for (1) Personal analysis, (2) Clinical work, (3) Supervision, (4) Didactic seminars, (5) Means of assessing progression, (6) Whether there have been past changes in training, and (7) Whether there is regular reflection on the training system's effectiveness.

Overall Atmosphere in the Training Institute

The overall atmosphere of the institute in terms of its morale, its viability, and its effective functioning form the backdrop and set the tone and parameters for the control analysis and the supervisions. For example, an institute's need to graduate analysts, to avoid candidate dissatisfactions, and to avoid confronting complicated pedagogical issues head-on may exert overt or covert pressure to "pass" the candidate and to overlook or downplay problems. In contrast, an institute may be organized in such a way that candidates do not graduate quickly or easily.

Policies About Supervision

Another factor that significantly affects the supervisory situation is the place and importance of the individual supervisor's assessment within the institute's progression procedures. In some institutes, the supervisor's judgments are highly influential and the sole determinant of progression and graduation. In other places, the supervisor's judgments are taken into account along with other opinions and evaluations. The supervisor may not get support for his or her judgments about the candidate if these differ from a prevailing view or from the judgment of other supervisors, instructors, or special committees. In general, candidates can be overidealized or underappreciated by the larger group, and these attitudes can impinge upon the supervisor's mind. Another difference among institutes which influences the supervisor's mindset is whether or not supervisors share their reports with each other.

Criteria for Progression

Connected to these influences are the differences that arise from the institutional criteria for progression and graduation, and whether

43

they are spelled out or not. In many cases, supervisors may follow their own inner criteria without having clearly agreed-upon or
articulated criteria from the training institution to serve as a guide.

Policies Around Personal "Training" Analyses

A frequent dilemma in supervisors' minds seems to be rooted in
their conflicts about addressing candidates' emotional problems and
blocks. The training analysis is set up to address these problems. Yet
institutes vary widely in their requirements for the training analysis,
for example, in how long candidates are required to be in analysis
before they can begin classes or a control case. In some cases, supervisors confronted a situation in which they experienced problems
in the supervised analysis as arising primarily from candidates who
were no longer in analysis or had a truncated, terminated analysis.
In such instances, supervisors felt helpless and alone, without institutional support.

The Working Party groups could see that the mind of the supervisor and indeed the whole atmosphere of the supervisory sessions
had become affected by such problems. In one case, for example,
the candidate who had interrupted two analyses seemed to have no
faith in the analytic process. The supervisor felt that the candidate
subtly rejected all his technical and theoretical suggestions. At the
same time, the supervisor was facing the fact that this advanced candidate was likely to be graduated by their institute. This supervisor
became mired in a sense of hopelessness and paralysis, a hopelessness that mirrored the candidate's doubts about psychoanalysis. As
has been documented in the literature on supervision, supervisors
vary widely in their philosophies of how to handle such personal
problems in candidates. Some steer clear of addressing the problems
while others make the supervisory session more like an analytic session by directly analyzing the candidate's countertransferences.

Relationships With Colleagues

A common, but not often openly acknowledged, external pressure related to the institutional setting is the supervisor's feelings
about the candidate's analyst who is a colleague at the institute.
This problem was also noted by Lebovici (1970), Haesler (1993), and
Skolnikoff (1997). The training analyst may be a friend or a political

foe, or may value different theoretical or technical positions. Such feelings about the training analyst can and often do enter supervisors' minds. Similarly, in institutes whose candidates are in analysis with training analysts from other institutes, there may be unconscious rivalries and/or different theoretical and educational climates. These reactions may operate as strong but unconscious influences on the supervisor's attitudes toward the candidate and the candidate's work (Kernberg, 2010).

Conflicts With Being Evaluators

Although less studied, we contend that the institutional requirement that supervisors serve as evaluators of candidates' progress is an omnipresent and often unacknowledged source of anxiety and conflict for supervisors (Junkers et al., 2008). The supervisor is first and foremost an analyst, and as such, he or she has been trained in a particular and unique way to suspend judgment of patients. When asked to supervise, the analyst assumes the roles of both educator and evaluator, and is often uncomfortable with these roles (Driver, 2008). From our Working Party findings, we concluded that supervisors may not fully appreciate the extent to which the role of the supervisor as a resonating, containing (good) object may be felt to conflict with an evaluative, limit-setting (bad) role. Faced with this conflict, which may be unconscious, supervisors may find it much easier to say what they think about the patient's dynamics or what to do technically than make important and life-changing judgments such as "Is this candidate ready or not ready to graduate?" We have seen supervisors' unwillingness to provide explicit assessments manifest itself in many ways – in a failure to talk to the supervisee clearly about his or her problems, for instance, or to be definite in making judgments about inadequacies. These reluctances are not always conscious and are often rationalized.

Another potential source of such indirectness on the part of supervisors is an unconscious investment in being idealized by candidates; these colleagues may prefer to leave the task of conveying critical comments to other members of the faculty, such as progression committee members. Consciously they may believe their roles as educators will be compromised by directly conveying evaluative comments, even though they do so in reports. Although the supervisee's vulnerability (as the less experienced member of the dyad who is being evaluated) has been emphasized in the literature, we found that supervisors felt vulnerable to being judged by colleagues, including the supervisee's analyst, or overruled in votes taken by the institute (Berman, 2000) or by the group in the Working Party.

Containment Function of the Group and the Institution

In their close examination of supervisory material, the authors were fascinated to find that these complex projections and identifications that bounced around among patient, candidate, and supervisor (and also in the Working Party group) occurred *in every supervision* that was subject to scrutiny. In certain cases, we found ourselves spontaneously referring to the disturbance in the supervisory dyad as "infection" because it could permeate supervisors' minds silently and without their knowledge.[1] While countertransference was at play to some degree in all clinical presentations, this did not always pose a serious or long-acting interference, especially when recognized by the supervisor. It also seemed to permeate the atmosphere in the group as they listened to the material. Sometimes the candidate and supervisor shared the same blind spot, while at other times they replicated a sadomasochistic interaction in the analysis in a subtle manner unbeknownst to both. These dynamics were similar to, but more complicated than, the "parallel process" described in the literature. A common denominator was the supervisor's and the candidate's inability to contain and metabolize the prevailing anxiety of the moment. *We were struck by how supervisors, in their roles as teacher, mentor, and especially as evaluator, were often not prepared to perceive, feel, or think about such strong emotions.* They most often strive to be objective educators, even if paradoxically they also routinely and consciously try to use emotions to understand the analytic material being presented. Supervisors believe that they are supposed to *know, to be the "expert."* This expectation then sets up a situation in which they may see themselves as exempt from unconscious pressures, which adds to a resistance to examine their supervisory work and can lead to a narcissistic vulnerability. As a profession, having discarded the myth of the "objective" analyst, we are freer to watch for countertransferential interferences (such as strong negative affects or gratifications from an idealizing

46

transference) and to seek a consultation in case of an impasse. However, in our role as supervisors, we have had resistance in recognizing and making use of our countertransferences and seeking consultations for our supervisory work (Mayman, 1976; Sandler, 1976; Martin et al., 1978; Teitelbaum, 1990; Frawley-O'Dea & Sarnat, 2001; Watkins, 2011).

We suspect that these "infections" noted earlier are phenomena that occur when boundaries are more permeable. In the conceptual terms of projective identification and container/contained processes that imply increased permeability of boundaries between self and other, it is understandable that the origin of countertransferences may be difficult to determine. Thus, they seem like "infections" that have no clear origin in patient, in analyst, or in supervisor. Yet, often in the exploratory discussions of a Working Party group, discernable dynamics related to known trauma and unbearable affects in the patient, and observable limitations in the supervisee, were at play when a supervisor lost clarity of thought about the case or judgment about the supervisee.

Weinstein et al. (2009), in close process monitoring of supervisory sessions, have found that shifts in modes of supervisory-supervisee interaction[2] signaled anxiety in one or both participants and reflected attempts at "mutual affect regulation occurring in the supervisory relationship" (p. 1392). They recommended close process monitoring to identify countertransferential lapses such as "lack of affective attunement, avoidance of uncomfortable or disturbing affects and collusion to overlook problematic areas" (p. 1396).

Our clinical examples show that countertransferences are evoked in the supervisor *in the present* about the candidate, or the candidate/patient dyad. As these examples demonstrate, we found that in every case these countertransferences interfered to some degree with the evaluation and supervisory process, but also that some sources of the disturbances could be comprehended through group discussion. Therefore, the Working Party moderators and consultants who reviewed reports of the group discussions and the supervisors' material in detail (summarized in the following case examples) conclude that to open the supervisory dyad to a "third" can facilitate and support good observation and evaluation. Through its policies and procedures, the training program can serve function in various ways.

47

Case Examples of the Variety of Supervisory Countertransferences ("Infection")

Example One: Institutional Impingement
and Parallel or Reverberating Processes

The supervisor presented to the End of Training Evaluation group (ETE) a candidate who was post-seminars and treating a middle-aged depressed woman. She described the candidate as hardworking, dedicated, and earnest with obsessional and intellectualizing tendencies. The candidate's patient, Ms. C., mother of two adult children and unhappily married, came to treatment with the goal of "finding her voice." The patient presented with a history of trauma, including abuse, sexual molestation, and painful losses. The supervisor reported to the ETE group that the candidate showed difficulty empathizing with Ms. C's frustration and deep pain. The supervisor observed that the candidate talked too much in the analytic hours, often in an authoritative and parental way, appearing robotic and formulaic as she attended to content and surface. In supervision, the candidate seemed to be "tone deaf," reading from her process notes and then taking meticulous notes on supervisory feedback. Following supervisory meetings, the candidate intervened in subsequent sessions with Ms. C. based on what she had just learned in supervision in an undigested way.[3] The supervisor struggled with frustration about not being able to reach the candidate emotionally; despite a wish to get through to her, she instead found herself backing away. The candidate confided to the supervisor that the patient reminded her of her own fragile mother. This kind of communication from a candidate about personal difficulties is noted elsewhere in the literature as deepening the transference of the supervisee to the supervisor, but ignores the parallel deepening of the supervisor's countertransference.

Initially, after hearing the supervisory process, the ETE group felt similarly discouraged about its capacity to help the supervisor and pessimistic about the candidate's capacity to function as an analyst. These feelings in a kind of parallel process receded as the supervisory countertransferences (feeling frustrated, helpless, critical, and holding back) were discussed by the group and understood as signals of traumatic experience, conflict, and defenses against them enacted within the patient-candidate dyad and echoed in the supervisor's withdrawal. The supervisor came to recognize more explicitly that both she and the candidate were experiencing the supervisory situation as dangerous, with the potential for feeling and acting upon strong disturbing emotions linked to the patient's experiences of abuse, sexual molestation, and loss. That is, the candidate consciously felt she might hurt the patient and unconsciously feared being hurt by her. A similar dynamic characterized the supervisory dyad. With the help of the group, the supervisor re-found *her* voice and more clearly recognized and articulated her complex identifications with both the patient's and the candidate's sadism and dissociated traumatic fears of intrusion, criticism, and abandonment. The complicated set of unconscious communications that reverberated among the three parties in this case cannot easily be captured by the term "parallel process."

The discussion also brought to light an institutional pressure to graduate candidates quickly (once they reached a certain level of seniority regardless of their level of competency), which might have contributed to the candidate's and supervisor's shared frustration and sense of urgency. The fact that the candidate needed this supervisor's approval to apply for graduation contributed to the intensity of the sadomasochistic dynamics in the supervisory situation. The situation of being evaluated by the supervisor intensified this candidate's strict superego and her perception of the supervisor as sadistic and withholding permission to graduate. This is one of many examples in the reported supervisions when a candidate needed more work in his or her own analysis. Speculating further, we can see how the candidate's early situation in relation to a fragile mother might have engendered pressure to grow up fast. That experience echoed in the supervisory dyad and found symbolic expression in institutional procedures that were then experienced as impingement.

Example 2: Institutional Impingement and the Supervisor's Idealizing Transference to Supervisee

The supervisor presented an advanced candidate, whom she introduced as an experienced psychotherapist with extensive theoretical knowledge. The patient, Mr. E., had a history of difficulties in relationships, including his current relationship. His past relationships involved triangular jealousies and infidelity. The analysis had been interrupted twice previously: once, when the patient relocated for several months for employment, and then again, because the analyst took a short leave for personal reasons. In one of supervisory sessions presented, the candidate had a critical tone and made some judgmental comments in response to the patient's mentioning that his girlfriend wanted a baby. While the candidate observed the fact that she had been critical of the patient, she did not appear to be curious about the meaning of her enactment or motivated to reflect on it. Similarly, the supervisor noticed, but did not discuss with the candidate, the fact that the candidate was enacting without reflecting.

With the help of the group, the supervisor realized that her defensive idealization of this candidate's knowledge of theory had compromised her ability to appreciate the candidate's defensive intellectualization and difficulty with intimacy. After the group discussion, the supervisor also realized that she, the candidate, and the patient were all backing away from their parallel anxiety about the patient's baby not having a good-enough mother. The supervisor also was struggling with her own deeper worries about the candidate's being a good-enough analyst and herself being a good-enough supervisor. Compounding the dynamics of the treatment and supervision, this institute's policy of only requiring two years of supervision limited the possibilities of exploring intimacy in both the supervision and in the analysis. The supervisor's not addressing the candidate's judgmental attitude may be another example of a conflict between being an understanding supervisor of clinical process and an evaluator of the candidate's progress.

Example 3: Institutional Impingement and
the Supervisor's Identification With a Patient

The supervisor presented an advanced candidate who had entered training with little psychotherapy experience and from a previous professional background that raised questions for some members of the faculty about his ability to become an analyst. The candidate was treating a highly traumatized and deprived middle-aged man, Mr. D., who had suffered at the hands of a psychotic mother and an unavailable father. Mr. D. grew up in a setting in which he was exposed to sexual overstimulation and physical danger, and had a history of transvestitism. The supervisor felt that the candidate was ready to graduate but had some lingering reservations that the progression committee might not agree with his assessment. In the supervisory sessions that the supervisor presented to the group, the candidate was able to self-supervise (for example, asking himself the meaning of his busily turning away from the patient before the patient left the consultation room at the end of each session).

The group observed that the supervisor trusted that the candidate was motivated to go to deeper and darker places and that he had a developing theory of therapeutic action that guided him. The supervisor conveyed to the group that the treatment was characterized by a sense of containment and safety because the danger was articulated and addressed in the transference/countertransference. As this candidate was discussed further within the Working Party group, the supervisor became much more certain in his own mind about the candidate's readiness to graduate. The supervisor became aware that his anxieties were about what members of his institute (who had previously expressed some doubts about this candidate's analytic ability) would think of him, rather than about the candidate. The group in this instance served as a container for the supervisor's anxiety about the candidate's readiness, based in his worry about the faculty not judging the candidate as ready to graduate, and hence judging him as well. In this instance, the supervisory limit setting and evaluating functions were projected onto the progression committee. Additional pressure was added to the system by a candidate that does not fit a typical mold.

Example 4: Institutional Impingement and Parallel Process

The supervisor was a relatively newly appointed supervising analyst who presented a supervision that was problematic for him. The supervision had been proceeding for three years and was the candidate's second case. The candidate had showed strong ambivalence towards training. In fact, he had interrupted his training analysis. The initial complaints of this patient, who was depressed and suffered from low self-esteem, were that he was too reliant on others' opinions and ideas. He seemed to be searching for an identity, both in his struggles with his chosen career and in his relationships with women. He had a history of difficulties with his alcoholic father from whom he was alienated.

The supervisor described how the candidate found it hard to intervene with the patient in any way. The candidate's fear to intervene intensified after his first case terminated unilaterally. The candidate

51

often became judgmental about this patient's inability to progress in his studies. The supervisor tried to help the candidate understand the patient's problems psychoanalytically, sharing with the supervisee his ideas that the patient identified with his father's failures and was afraid to surpass him (which, by implication, was a dynamic in the transference). The candidate agreed with this formulation but was not able to integrate this understanding into his interventions in the sessions. The group was able to perceive the supervisor's ideas about what a "good enough" analysis was, and how he tried to impart his ideas to the candidate both directly and in his supervisory style. He stressed the importance of interpretation, tolerating affects, and the use the countertransference, largely by modeling these in his functioning as a supervisor, but the supervisee did not seem to identify with the supervisor in these ways.

The patient tended to intellectualize about psychoanalysis and philosophy. In spite of this, he came regularly and appeared dependent on the analyst, although he had difficulty keeping up with his payments and often came late. The candidate too began to come late and not pay the supervisor promptly. The group was struck by the parallel process in these enactments around the frame. In listening to the material, they became aware of how they, in identification with the supervisor, began to feel hopeless and lethargic. The group also agreed that the candidate identified with the patient. Both had difficulty in facing feelings and finding a distance from which to observe the analytic process and their feelings. The patient was inhibited and full of shame; the candidate seemed even more inhibited. A group countertransference and counter-identification emerged as the participants repeatedly confused patient and candidate in their comments. In terms of countertransference, the group speculated that the supervisor may have switched off his supervisory function at times as the candidate switched off his own analyzing function. Members also conjectured that his subtle withdrawal may have been evident in the sense of boredom experienced by the group in discussing the supervision. The boredom may also have reflected the sense of hopelessness that the supervisor and analyst shared.

What became increasingly clear was that the problem was a personal one within the supervisee, who needed further analysis. Moreover, this particular institute did not have a clear administrative policy about guidelines for the candidates' analyses. The supervisor felt inhibited about bringing up the issue of personal problems and personal analysis, both with the candidate and the institute, given the additional pressure of candidates' presence in progression meetings. With the help of group discussion, the supervisor felt more empowered to speak directly to the candidate about his problems that were interfering with his ability to analyze.

This situation is not uncommon. In another institute in which the supervisor felt that the candidate's personal problems were interfering with the candidate's being able to deal with sexual material, the candidate had also interrupted her analysis. In this institute, the situation was further complicated because the supervisors did not share reports about the candidates they have in common so that a supervisor did not know if the candidate's problem was unique to the particular case or more general.

Case 5: Supervisor's Countertransference and Relationships With Colleagues

A somewhat similar situation to that in the previous case characterized a supervisory situation presented at another meeting of a Working Party in another country, but with a much more senior supervisor, surer of herself and her place in the profession. The candidate was a young unmarried woman, who was beginning her first case. The supervisor felt that the candidate was very talented and sensitive. In contrast to the previous candidate, this candidate felt very enthusiastic about psychoanalysis, starting, according to the supervisor, with the fantasy that once the patient got into four times a week analysis after previous psychotherapy, everything would magically become easier and that his problems would lessen. The candidate was known to be feisty, independent, and questioning. The supervisor appreciated and seemed to identify with these qualities. However, she felt that the faculty of the institute was in disagreement about this young woman's potential – the female faculty all agreed with the supervisor, but the men were less than enthusiastic. The supervisor was angry about it. Moreover, the faculty's opinions about a given candidate carried weight. In this particular institute, compared to other institutes across the world, the faculty has a much bigger voice in deciding a candidate's progression and ultimate graduation; graduation is judged by candidates' case presentations to a "symposium" comprised of the whole faculty. In other institutes, in comparison, the decision, while made in a group, is much more strongly dependent on a smaller number of voices, especially those of the supervisors. Such unwelcome worries, rivalries, alliances, theoretical differences – unconscious and conscious – are expectable but rarely admitted, let alone spoken of, but of course infiltrate supervisors' minds.

The patient was a man who was stuck in life. Disappointed with his boss, he had quit a promising job. His girlfriend had left him, and deeply depressed, he kept himself at home. As an infant and toddler, he had suffered from genetic abnormalities and painful treatments that had to be administered by his mother. As a result, he had developed a very compliant, masochistic stance toward life and people. As revealed in the supervisor's discussions and the candidate's progress notes, the transference was characterized by overt compliance and need to please, with underlying unconscious anger and neediness. The patient's anger seemed to be expressed in his missing sessions frequently due to his debilitating depression and inertia.

Listening to the early supervisory sessions, the group noted and agreed with the supervisor's emphasis on the patient's unconscious and conflicted aggression. The emerging transference, evidenced in repeated anxious complaints from the patient that he was feeling worse and worse, conveyed a picture of an unhelpful, hurtful mother re-experienced and re-created within the analytic dyad. Much anger, of different sorts, seemed to bounce around patient, candidate, and supervisor. For the most part, however, the supervisor remained steady and calm, modeling in this and her nondirective and accepting attitude an analytic attitude.

Interesting patterns emerged in the supervision: the candidate often would begin a session by asking if the supervisor wanted to hear a dream of the patient. The supervisor would reply, "As you wish." Then the supervisee would present something else and never get to the dream. Some of the group thought the supervisee's waffling about what she should present to the supervisor might be an example of "parallel process." The patient consciously tried to please and submit, just as the candidate tried to gauge what the supervisor wanted to hear. Others were not at all sure what this behavior meant – was it wanting to please or some kind of teasing? It was clear, however, that the candidate was attached and trusting of the supervisor. She had picked her as supervisor especially because she wanted someone who was known in the institute to be "tough" but from whom she could learn a lot.

The candidate was quickly disabused of her fantasy of an easy transition from the psychotherapy to analysis as she was confronted with the patient's refrain about how painful the treatment and life were. The patient seemed regressed, crippled by depression and anxiety. Over time, however, the candidate was more and more able to be empathic toward the patient and to begin to deal with these "negative" transferences. The patient seemed totally ignorant of his mind (only his pain and his body) and unable to take in what his analyst was saying. As the treatment progressed over several months, the supervisor felt that the candidate was more ready to hear that she was frightened by the patient's anger and uncomfortable being the "bad object." (Supervisors differ widely in how they deal with such countertransferences in supervision. This supervisor simply pointed it out.) The group felt it was witnessing an inexperienced, but talented candidate blossoming with the help of the careful and sensitive hand of this supervisor, even within the six months of supervisory notes that were presented.

The supervisor confessed to an important and puzzling action on her part that, in a way, could be read as an exclamation mark to the whole presentation. She told the group that she had the habit of writing up these supervisory sessions, which she anticipated presenting, immediately after each session. She had written up nine supervisory sessions that spanned six months and several breaks. But she consciously postponed writing down the tenth session for several days to spend time visiting with her family – her children and grandchildren. When the supervisor returned to record the tenth and last session, it was totally gone from her mind! She could not remember anything at all about it. She could very well just have not told the group about this and presented nine sessions, which certainly provided more than ample material to discuss and no one would have been the wiser. But her openness prevailed since she knew this action on her part must have important meanings.

The group speculated that the forgetting did not have to do with the specific content of that last session, but somehow to the whole of the case and the supervisory situation. First, they noted that the theme of bad mother/good mother from the analysis was being played out in this way. The supervisor chose to be the "good" mother to her children. Then in keeping with the whole discussion, one member expressed the thought that this action could be taken as an expression of how the death drive was so prominent in the case.

That is, that the patient was seriously in danger of destroying himself and his life. Another participant pointed out the atmosphere in the supervisor's psychoanalytic society was pressing in on the supervisor, perhaps creating a need to escape it internally.

The next morning (the Working Parties usually meet two days in a row) the supervisor reported what came to her after her night's sleep and the discussion the afternoon before. With an awakened sense of conviction, she realized that she had been out of touch with the *erotic* in the case: the idea of "forbidden love," the patient's unconscious yearnings for the candidate, covered over in his acting out and the emphasis in all the theorizing about the case on his anger. Clearly the supervisor was fond of the candidate, a loved analytic daughter. In confirmation of the supervisor's insight, the leader of the group revealed she had woken up thinking about the case and slipped into a reverie with the old children's verse "he loves me/he loves me not" – or was it "she loves me, she loves me not?" – running through her head. Through this unconscious act of omission, the supervisor's attention was drawn to the idea that there was something important and powerful, and heretofore not conscious, that she was missing in this case and in herself – the erotic elements very much alive in the analytic dyad and the supervisory dyad.

Discussion and Summary

An effort to mine the Working Group material for expression of institutional influences reveals the hidden and embedded shape such influences may take. We have seen how these impingements become embroiled in the dynamics of the transference/countertransferences and unconscious communications that reverberate among all three participants: analysand, candidate, and supervisor. The institute, through its procedures and relationships, can help to provide a stabilizing and holding function for the supervisory situation and help the supervisor and candidate contain the strong emotions that arise there. The faculty can help to support and nourish each other in their educational and analytic functioning.

At times, however, the institute can falter in its function of containment. Institutional procedures can come alive and be experienced as uncomfortable encounters between supervisee and supervisor that diminish valued aspects of supervisor's authority. When the institute fails to provide clear policies about progression or personal analyses, as in several of these examples, the supervisor feels unsupported and thus less able to support and contain the supervisee. Institutional rivalries and disputes can shake the foundation of the supervisory setting and impinge on the supervisor's sense of balance and objectivity. In the last case, for example, we can observe how the supervisor's relationship with the other faculty in her institute became interwoven with her unconscious identifications and feelings about the supervisee.

In the pursuit of investigating institutional influences in analytic training, the ETE Working Party has considered cases with emphasis on the dynamics of clinical and technical issues from the viewpoint of the supervising analyst. Other papers written by the other participants of the triad may contain implied or embedded institutional influences. A recent example is by Broder (2020), written from the candidate's standpoint about the experience of a failed control case. Only after a long time did the institutional impingement in the form of complex fee regulations with powerful resonance within the supervisory triad emerge as a central issue. A second is a paper by Brown (2020) written to elaborate on field theory in the supervisory relationship. He describes his own experience as a psychoanalytic candidate treating an inhibited college student struggling with issues of moving on with his life. Both Brown and his supervisor shared their respective dreams which followed two significant events at their institute – a progression meeting and a graduation party – and demonstrated "coming of age" anxieties. In retrospect, Brown speculated that themes of rivalry and competition had permeated the supervisory atmosphere. The discussion of their dreams revealed shared unconscious anxieties that provided data about similar issues that had been stalling the analysis (Gerson, 2004). These findings point to the possibility of further research in several different directions.

Notes

1 The Working Party on Initiating Psychoanalysis reported that "affective storms" were the most robust finding in their qualitative research on the critical elements in the initial consultation (Reith, 2010). They later settled on the term "unconscious storms" (Reith et al., 2018).
2 The authors identified a moral mode, a therapeutic mode, an empirical mode, and a modeling mode of supervisor-supervisee interaction.
3 This is a good example of what has been called "supervisory lag."

Bibliography

Arlow, J. A. (1963). The supervisory situation. *Journal of the American Psychoanalytic Association, 11,* 576–594.

Baudry, F. D. (1993). The personal dimension and management of the supervisory situation with a special note on the parallel process. *Psychoanalytic Quarterly, 62,* 588–614.

Berman, E. (2000). Psychoanalytic supervision. *International Journal of Psychoanalysis, 81,* 273–290.

Bion, W. R. (1965). *Transformations.* Tavistock.

Broder, R. (2020, February). Low fee, rage, and countertransference: A parallel process [Paper presentation]. American Psychoanalytic Association, New York.

Brown, L. J. (2020, February). A field theory approach to supervision in child analysis [Paper presentation]. American Psychoanalytic Association, New York.

Caligor, L. (1981). Parallel and reciprocal processes in psychoanalytic supervision. *Contemporary Psychoanalysis, 17,* 1–27.

Doehrman, M. J. G. (1976). Parallel processes in supervision and psychotherapy. *Bulletin of the Menninger Clinic, 40,* 3–104.

Driver, C. (2008). Assessment in supervision: An analytic perspective. *British Journal of Psychotherapy, 24,* 328–342.

Ehrlich, L., Hanly, M., Kulish, N., Robinson, M., & Rothstein, A. (2017). Supervisory countertransferences and impingements in evaluating readiness for graduation: Always present, routinely under-recognized. *International Journal of Psychoanalysis, 98,* 491–516.

Ekstein, R., & Wallerstein, R. S. (1958). *The teaching and learning of psychotherapy.* International Universities Press.

Erlich-Ginor, M. (2010). The EPF Working Party on education: An overview. *EPF Bulletin, 64* (Supplement), 33–56.

Erlich, S., & Erlich-Ginor, M. (2018). Psychoanalytic training – Who is afraid of evaluation? *International Journal of Psychoanalysis, 99* (5), 1129–1143.

Frawley-O'Dea, M. G., & Sarnat, J. (2001). *The supervisory relationship: A contemporary psychodynamic approach.* Guilford Press.

Gediman, H. K., & Wolkenfeld, F. (1980). The parallelism phenomenon in psychoanalysis and supervision: Its reconsideration as a triadic system. *Psychoanalytic Quarterly, 49,* 243–255.

Gerson, S. (2004). The relational unconscious. *Psychoanalytic Quarterly, 73,* 63–98.

Haesler, L. (1993). Adequate distance in the relationship between supervisor and supervisee – The position of the supervisor between "teacher" and "analyst". *International Journal of Psychoanalysis, 74,* 547–555.

Hinze, E. (2013). Expanding the field: Clinical working party today. *International Journal of Psychoanalysis, 94*, 1194–1196.

Hinze, E. (2015). What do we learn in psychoanalytic training? *International Journal of Psychoanalysis, 96*, 755–771.

Hinze, I. (2014, March). End of training evaluation project [Paper presentation]. North American Working Party Meeting, New York.

Jacobs, D. (2001). Narcissism, eroticism, and envy in the supervisory relationship. *Journal of the American Psychoanalytic Association, 49*, 813–830.

Jaffe, L. (2001). Countertransference, supervised analysis, and psychoanalytic training requirements. *Journal of the American Psychoanalytic Association, 49*, 831–853.

Junkers, G., Tuckett, D., & Zachrisson, A. (2008). To be or not to be a psychoanalyst – How do we know a candidate is ready to qualify? Difficulties and controversies in evaluating psychoanalytic competence. *Psychoanalytic Inquiry, 28*, 288–308.

Kernberg, O. F. (2010). Psychoanalytic supervision: The supervisor's tasks. *Psychoanalytic Quarterly, 79*, 603–627.

Lebovici, S. (1970). Technical remarks on the supervision of psychoanalytic treatment. *International Journal of Psychoanalysis, 51*, 385–392.

Lester, E. P., & Robertson, B. M. (1995). Multiple interactive processes in psychoanalytic supervision. *Psychoanalytic Inquiry, 15*, 211–225.

Martin, G. C., Mayerson, P., Olsen, H. E., & Wiberg, J. L. (1978). Candidates' evaluation of psychoanalytic supervision. *Journal of the American Psychoanalytic Association, 26*, 407–424.

Mayman, M. (1976). Parallel processes in supervision and psychotherapy. *Bulletin of the Menninger Clinic, 40*, 1–8.

Mendelsohn, R. (2012). Parallel process and projective identification in psychoanalytic supervision. *Psychoanalytic Review, 99*, 297–314.

Miller, L., & Twomey, J. E. (1999). A parallel without a process. *Contemporary Psychoanalysis, 35*, 557–580.

Reith, B. (2010). The specific dynamics of initial interviews: Switching the level, or opening up a meaning space? *European Federation of Psychoanalysis: Bulletin, 64* (Supplement), 57–80.

Reith, B., Møller, M., Boots, J., Crick, P., Gibeault, A., Jaffè, R., Lagerlöf, S., & Vermote, R. (2018). *Beginning analysis: On the processes of initiating psychoanalysis.* Routledge.

Sandler, J. (1976). Countertransference and role-responsiveness. *International Review of Psycho-Analysis, 3*, 43–47.

Searles, H. F. (1986). The informational value of the supervisor's emotional experiences. In H. F. Searles (Ed.), *Collected papers on schizophrenia and related subjects* (pp. 157–176). Maresfield Library. (Original work published 1955).

Skolnikoff, A. Z. (1997). The supervisorial situation: Intrinsic and extrinsic factors influencing transference and countertransference themes. *Psychoanalytic Inquiry, 17*, 90–107.

Stimmel, B. (1995). Resistance to awareness of the supervisor's transferences with special reference to the parallel process. *International Journal of Psychoanalysis, 76*, 609–618.

Strean, H. S. (1991). Colluding illusions among analytic candidates, their supervisors, and their patients: A major factor in some treatment impasses. *Psychoanalytic Psychology, 8*, 403–414.

Target, M. (2001, March). Some issues in psychoanalytic training: An overview of the literature and some resulting observations [Paper presentation]. 2nd Joseph Sandler Research Conference, University College, London.

Teitelbaum, S. H. (1990). Supertransference. *Psychoanalytic Psychology, 7*, 243–258.

Tuckett, D. (2000). The EPF policy and objectives for the next four years. *EPF Bulletin, 54*, 111–118.

Tuckett, D. (2003). A ten-year European scientific initiative: Presidential address. *EPF Bulletin, 57*, 7–21.

Tuckett, D. (2005). Does anything go? *International Journal of Psychoanalysis, 86*, 31–49.

Watkins, C. E., Jr. (2011). Toward a tripartite vision of supervision for psychoanalysis and psychoanalytic psychotherapies: Alliance, transference-countertransference configuration, and real relationship. *Psychoanalytic Review, 98*, 557–590.

Weinstein, L. S., Winer, J. A., & Ornstein, E. (2009). Supervision and self-disclosure: Modes of supervisory interaction. *Journal of the American Psychoanalytic Association, 57*, 1379–1400.

Werbart, A. (2007). Utopic ideas of cure and joint exploration in psychoanalytic supervision. *International Journal of Psychoanalysis, 88*, 1391–1408.

Zaslavsky, J., Nunes, M. L., & Eizirik, C. L. (2005). Approaching countertransference in psychoanalytical supervision. *International Journal of Psychoanalysis, 86*, 1099–1131.

3

THE SPECIFICITY OF PSYCHOANALYTIC TREATMENT TODAY

Research by the Paris Group

Serge Frisch and Martine Sandor-Buthaud and the members of the Paris Group: Jan Abram, Leopoldo Bleger, Catherine Desvignes, Marie-France Dispaux-Ducloux, Yvette Dorey, Erika Kittler, Fabienne Fillion, Serge Frisch, Lila Hoijman, Matthew Mc Ardle, Diana Messina, Luc Michel, Martine Sandor, Andrea Scardovi, Ronnie Shaw, Philippe Valon

Introduction

The Working Party (WP) on the Specificity of Psychoanalytic Treatment Today from its inception was part of the Research Program of the European Psychoanalytic Federation (EPF). This research group has developed a research method to make it possible to identify certain specific elements of a psychoanalytic treatment, and the unfolding of a treatment, to serve as a "tool" for the investigation and assessment of the treatment's evolution and its effects.

The initial idea was to use free association, i.e. the fundamental psychoanalytic rule as defined by Freud, as a working tool in our clinical groups, in order to carry out a way of researching the specific aspects of the analytic process. A large part of our work, in fact, concerned the setting up of this research method. Thus our "Specificity methodology" became the subject of research which included an investigation of its tools, and its epistemology. The framework of our research took shape as we progressed in exploring our questions.

DOI: 10.4324/9781032656311-3

How could we apply free association to listen, as freely as possible, to the presented work of analysis and analyst in the Specificity groups? How could we listen and think about what occurs when a group of analysts associate to clinical material? What could this possibly teach us about the analytic process and its method?

The method of the research was initially developed in Europe in small clinical groups scheduled in the days preceding the EPF and IPA congress. The small clinical groups are made up of between twelve and fifteen analysts of various languages and analytic cultures working for a day and a half on the same clinical material. The method of working was inspired by the work of Norman and Salomonsson (2005) and Donnet (2005). It is based on the narrative of an analytic session in a group of analysts and the hypothesis an analogy between what emerges in the group and the process of the encounter between the patient and the analyst. The group listens to the clinical session and then "treats" both the analyst's counter-transference and the unknown aspects of the patient's transference. Analyzing the processes underlying the inter-analytic exchanges in our clinical groups during the discussion of clinical material presented by an experienced psychoanalyst thus becomes the core of our research. The method proposed to the participants to work with the clinical material is the one used internally by the analyst during the session. Wondering about what happens in groups using this method facilitates an opportunity to research the functioning of the analytic method, and the process that is set in motion particularly in the inner life of the analyst during each session when he treats and transforms clinical material.

Clinical exchanges, especially in an international context, are an important and productive experience of psychoanalysis today. The question of the specificity of psychoanalysis is a central issue for the entire psychoanalytic community. New economic and cultural conditions have reinforced resistance from both the external world as well as internal resistance concerning psychoanalysts' confidence in psychoanalysis as a form of treatment. This question is also part of the controversy with psychotherapies and the application of psychoanalysis to "new pathologies." Some analysts, for example, consider it not possible to respond to these new pathologies by concepts shaped by 19th century scientific thought.

The analytic approach and technique has evolved since its beginning. The participants of the clinical groups we offer come from different countries, continents and analytical approaches. Beyond the abundance of differences in contemporary psychoanalysis, we consider that the fundamental rule of free association and its counterpart, the free floating listening of the analyst, constitute a common basis. The participants of our groups tell us, and as participants of the research we know this ontologically, that the Specificity method in groups reaffirms the power of the fundamental rule and facilitates a "renewed experience" of it. It has led us to many questions and developments which we aim to account for in this chapter.

The Birth and History of the Specificity of Psychoanalytical Treatment Today

The WP Specificity of Psychoanalytic Treatment Today (SPTT) was created in 2006 by Evelyne Séchaud, who was at that time president of the EPF. Since 2009, WP Specificity has spread to North America, Latin America, and recently, Australia. In each region, it has developed independently, exploring different avenues, both in the clinical and in the research groups. The initial idea was to build on the couple-based psychoanalytic technique that was led by free association and listening in equal measure, as Freud had painstakingly developed. Europeans followed the idea to conduct research that employs the psychoanalytic method rather than enlisting rules and methods applied in other disciplines.

The aim is not to judge what the analyst does or whether what they do is psychoanalytic or psychotherapeutic work. Rather, our project is to reflect, without prior knowledge and as much as possible without hypotheses and "purposive ideas" (*représentations-buts*; *Zielvorstellungen*), on the specificity of psychoanalysis based on clinical material that includes patients who present non-neurotic psychic functioning as seen today in our practices, while taking into account the gap between practice and theory. It is indeed psychoanalysis "today" that we are dealing with, treated in the face of challenges and questions that current conditions impose.

The title given to this Working Party reflects the spirit of the desired research. The association of the terms "specificity" and "today" could, at first sight, lead to confusion. Indeed, specificity is that "which presents an original and exclusive characteristic" (TLF Dictionary, 2004). But, as Leopoldo Bleger (2009) points out, specificity, i.e., here, specificity of psychoanalysis, could not then vary according to circumstances or history nor be linked to a temporal condition. However, the "today" of the title contradicts the idea that the specificity or specificities of psychoanalysis would be immutable. It is a question of thinking about what the specificity (or the specificities) of psychanalysis is according to what analysts consider to be "psychoanalytical treatment" today. The whole point of this title is to contain this contradiction and complementarity which, generative of elaborations, circumscribe a field of relevant questions.

What the specificity of psychoanalysis today reveals is precisely the present conditions of its exercise. It is not a question of advocating modifications of psychoanalysis according to today's social pressures and cultural difficulties, but rather, following step by step the way psychoanalysis evolves while remaining specific. "Today" also refers to the "multicultural situation" of psychoanalysis today in which each participant in our clinical groups brings something from their own original analytic culture. This diversity can be actualized in the material of our groups.

Let us now come to the term "treatment" which is to be understood in its double meaning of therapeutic modality and transformation of the unconscious material. In this sense, the "result" of the analytic process is evaluated by the characteristics of psychic productivity so that "treatment" also means process, change, evolution, and transformation of psychic material. In our groups, we submit the presented clinical material to analytical processing by the participants' free associations, and seek to identify the processes that are triggered and the pathways that these processes use, as well as those they instigate in the group.

Treatment is also the way in which a psychoanalyst "treats" all the elements of the material conveyed to him, starting with the phenomenon of his own personal psychic experiences. This position is not new, but taking into account the way in which the analyst transforms his own psychic experiences is today certainly more recognized than it was in the early days of psychoanalysis. Specificity would therefore be essentially the way a psychoanalyst is thinking about the clinical situation, following the impact and the intensity of what has to be dealt with, as well as the way in which they manage it. The polysemy of the term "treatment" bears witness to the richness of language and the pleasure that the analyst can have in playing with words and their meaning, which invokes interesting reflections on the characters and modalities of what constitutes an analytic narrative, whether oral or written.

The Epistemological Foundations

Reflecting on epistemology, present in the founding moments of our group from the outset, has become increasingly important over time. Research in psychoanalysis can take several forms: clinical research, conceptual research, and empirical research. Daniel Widlöcher (2007) distinguishes between research "on" psychoanalysis and research "in" psychoanalysis. Research "on" psychoanalysis, most often carried out by non-analysts, uses instruments external to psychoanalysis, for example, evaluation grids derived from psychology, psychiatry, or sociology. Research "in" psychoanalysis is carried out exclusively by psychoanalysts because it applies the psychoanalytic method on material collected in an analyzing situation which only an analyst can implement. It is from such a clinical approach that all the major theoretical models proposed by Freud originated, and it is on the basis of the clinical approach that the controversies arising from these models developed. This approach, which is based exclusively on a clinical approach and reflection on its after-effects, has the advantage of a methodological coherence applied to the very particular unconscious material which cannot be approached directly. Freud asserted that unconscious phenomena were almost inaccessible outside the analytic method.

Theories are evolving models, not objects that are frozen forever. There are two tendencies in current research: one that wants to reduce the gap between theory and practice, and one that believes that this gap is essential and vital for psychoanalysis. For those who hold the latter position, as we do, the tension between practice and theory would be seen as a source of productivity and creativity. It allows us to use the theory not as an immutable knowledge but as an apperception of an unconscious phenomenon. Donnet (1995, p. 298) states this point when writing that there is "an active penetration of the unconscious into the theory that is supposed to represent it." These two conceptions of knowledge overlap with that of the theory of the unconscious and lead to opposite positions. It even seems to us that this gap is, for us, the very place where Freudian research is active.

65

In order to understand our research references, it is important to recall the complex definition of psychoanalysis given by Freud (1955/1922, p. 235) which articulates three levels by distinguishing between each. Psychoanalysis is:

1. A process of investigation of unconscious psychic processes, which are otherwise hardly accessible. This process is that of the free association of ideas.
2. A method of treatment of psychic disorders, which is based on this investigation.
3. A theorizing process which organizes the knowledge gained from this practical experience, which in turn is inspired by it.

For Freud, it would therefore be impossible to separate the process of clinical investigation of mental disorders from research. Freud places in first place this definition of the investigative method that allows unconscious psychic processes to be discovered and cannot be discovered otherwise, and he places theory in third and last place. Starting from existing concepts and theories without taking into account research about the method seems to us to be of a different nature.

Our method is fueled by this specificity of the Freudian method of research which has just been recalled, i.e., the establishment of a way of thinking, of deducing, and of making hypotheses about which analysts all over the world can debate. This is why the way of treating the clinical material presented in the groups and of listening to what emerges from this treatment becomes both the object and the result of the research.

From an epistemological point of view, there are therefore two possible pathways: either the research is based on preliminary hypotheses which is a question of verifying, or, the findings of the research result from the recurrence of the phenomena which appear in different clinical presentations. The second path is the one chosen by the idea of Specificity. Specificity is an "action research." The method is conceived as "the possibility of reconstructing the pathway one has taken, without having a clear and conscious awareness of it" (Lalande, 1991, p. 624).

Our objective is to remain as open as possible to, on the one hand, listening to what will emerge in the group's associative process, and, on the other hand, listening to the analogy between what emerges in the group and the process of the encounter between the patient and the analyst.

> In such a way that the research leads itself without a prior 'purposive aim' of the goal. It is in the *après-coup* that it seems possible to us to try to restore the method, i.e., the pathway followed with the feeling that this is indeed a proper analytic research.
>
> (Donnet, unpublished text)

The *Dispositif*

We have gradually established a way of working we refer to as the *dispositif* or modus operandi.[1] Its implementation and the understanding of what was at stake were the central object of our research, and its modifications are the consequence, through the *après coup* (*Nachträglichkeit* or deferred action) of the previous experiments and their elaborations.

Each method constructs its object and its specific approach to this object, which it defines in a singular way.

We propose to a group of analysts, all IPA analysts and candidates, to "treat" the clinical material presented by an experienced colleague just as each analyst treats the clinical material during a session in a treatment. That is to say, to let the material penetrate as they allow themselves to associate and listen in a free-floating way. Through this analytic way of listening to the material, with the stress on how each analyst responds emotionally, they will start to hypothesize on the functioning of the transference in the treatment and on the psychic reality of the patient. This work is mediated by the group and is based on group processes but is not a work that is centered on the analysis of group processes.

We propose to work over two days, which introduces one night into the approach, in order to open up a dream space. The term "scansion" is used in Lacan's work, meaning a pause in the rhythm of analytic work. One night constitutes the pause.

In the congresses of the EPF and the IPA we organize several clinical groups. We begin the meeting with the chair and co-chair of the WPSPTT, all the presenters, moderators, and reporters reviewing the general instructions and the specific work of each role. At the plenary, which follows this first meeting, all the participants are present. Then, each group meets separately. We end with a final plenary meeting. In addition to the participating analysts (from ten to fifteen) and the presenter, each group has two moderators and an observer-reporter. In the two plenary meetings and in the instructions given by the moderators in each group we remind everyone about the rules of confidentiality, and we stress the importance to respect them. Apart from the ethical necessity, always present in our work as analysts, confidentiality is an indispensable condition for liberating a sense of freedom when participating.

At the beginning of each group, the moderators also give to the participants the instructions and operating rules of our method: they are told the temporal structure of the model; they are asked to associate as freely as possible whatever comes to mind while listening to each reported session; and then they are asked to speak as spontaneously as possible, without selection and without value judgment, to give the thoughts, impressions, or feelings that have arisen in them and those that arise as the other participants speak. This clearly evokes the fundamental analytic rule and facilitates certain associations and thoughts that slowly, sometimes confusedly, emerge in each person and in relation to others.

The presenter prepares three or four written consecutive sessions of an "analytic week" with a patient without reporting anything about the anamnesis or the history of the analysis. He or she plunges the participants directly into a session without them knowing the gender or age of the patient. After each reported session, the group is invited to associate while the presenter remains silent and does not answer any direct questions that could be put to him. On indication of the moderators, the presenter reads the first session which will be followed by an exchange among the participants. At the request of the moderators again, he will read the second session, and the associative work of the group will follow. Likewise, for the next sessions. The presenter will be invited to speak only at the end of the second day, which the presenter and the group know from the beginning.

The participants are invited not to reflect intellectually but rather to suspend their judgment and to associate on the material presented to them. The participants associate not only on the patient and the verbal exchanges reported, but also on the interventions of the other participants. The work is done on the basis of the material heard and then gradually becomes an associative fabric to which each participant contributes their thoughts, ideas, and hypotheses. In this way, a work of thought is done, a "weaving of thought" to use the beautiful formula of Norman and Salomonsson (2005), a weaving close to the thought of the dream more than a secondary process work of reflection. This associative group work seems to us to be close to the analytic functioning and to what happens inside the analyst and between the analyst and his analysand. It is this work which can allow one to hear the unconscious dynamics, in a treatment and here in the material presented.

Participating in Specificity groups is a very special personal and group experience. Suspending judgment and allowing time for reflection, or even uncertainty in a group can be difficult for the participants and can cause uncertainty and anxiety in them. However, many of the participants also express that the feeling and experience they have in these groups is the stuff of analysis, and what psychoanalytic practice is all about. Some who come to work in the groups on a regular basis talk about coming to have "an analytic-reminder-shot." In other words, the experience constitutes a reminder about the strength of the analytic method, about the strength of associating and the interactivity of transferences, as well as a kind of incentive, or even permission, to hold onto those fundamentals of psychoanalysis more firmly.

The exchange among the participants in the group seems to us to tend to go through three stages: the one in which they try to objectify the functioning of the patient; secondly, there is a slide towards a certain subjectivation that finally becomes an exchange that focuses on intersubjectivity, focused on the latent more than on the manifest. Gradually, the material is no longer the narrative offered by the presenter, but rather, the narrative together with its effects on the group, and participants get used to and accept thinking aloud in front of others and working with their own reactions to the material, as each analyst does in the privacy of the sessions with his patients. Our *dispositif* makes it possible to perceive the hidden force emanating both from the patient's story and from the analytic situation itself. It is by this means that it becomes accessible, just as free association makes unconscious movements perceptible and accessible through interpretation.

Some may fear that this method may be tilted towards a form of transgression, wild analysis, group therapy, or group dynamics. These risks exist in the most banal of seminars. Our attention takes these dangers particularly into account, and we have increasingly emphasized this part of the function of the moderators, who need to be permanently vigilant in order to maintain the listening conditions of the associations as closely as possible to the analytic method. This last point highlights that we have gradually developed our method of listening and that we have increasingly grasped the fundamental function of moderators in these groups, which is to ensure that exchanges remain in an associative mode.

One could also issue the objection that using "free association" should stay specific and exclusive to psychoanalytic treatment. But, in our view, "free association" as a thinking activity is not only specific to the fundamental rule in psychoanalytic treatment, but is a characteristic of psychic functioning. On the other hand, what seems to us to be specific to psychoanalysis, and which is at the foundation of its method, is the particular type of listening to "free" association. The fundamental rule of free association is a result of the type of listening and a consequence of it (Roussillon, 2009).

The study of what is happening in our groups has allowed us to see that listening to the reading of a session sets in motion, unbeknownst to the participants, a reproduction of what had taken place during the session itself. In this instance, we have chosen not to focus on the situation itself, as is done in other fields, but to examine something else that can be referred to as a focus on the displacement onto another that becomes like a "replica." It is not a carbon copy, nor a re-duplication, but rather the staging of issues at stake in the treatment, as well as the possible revelation of processes that are specific to the analyst's work. This hypothesis would perhaps make it possible to get around the methodological problems posed today by research and evaluation in psychoanalysis.

> By exporting a tiny part of the treatment in such a setting – which is already a transgressive gesture – the responses from the participants create a sounding board and carry out a work of transformation and displacement by working on "the loom of the transference"; they tackle the task of its treatment, seeking to appreciate its "state" and what it conveys, discovering and rediscovering the succession of "displacements," "shifts" and "remnants" that are not in what is being said; a sequence of the analysis presented, but also in the very presentation of the sequence of analysis.
>
> (Dorey, 2010, p 84)

In her paper, Jan Abram (2014) describes the process created in the group as an inter-analytic mirror. She shows clearly in the group the dynamics of reproduction and of replica, and also the gaps, of which we will discuss later in this chapter.

This phenomenon that we have called replica, in the sense of the aftershock of an earthquake, appears clearly in the example that will be explained later in more depth, where two groups of the Specificity WP working on different clinical materials each reacted to the same intrusive external noise, the reactions being inflected by the dynamics at work in the case presented. As we will see, each of the groups replicated this dynamic in its reaction.

In our *dispositive*, until the end of the second day, the group works and associates while the presenter, as noted earlier, remains silent. The time when the presenter is allowed to speak is not conceived by us as a time of unveiling, but rather as another moment until the end of that of the group process. It is not so much a question of obtaining information about the patient or the treatment, as if it could give an "objective" confirmation of the group's elaborative work, but more about continuing the process by integrating the work that took place inside the presenter while he remained silent and listened in a free-floating way to the work of the group. It is astonishing to often hear the presenter say how much the group has reconstituted the patient, their history, and the transferential dynamics at work in the treatment. The presenter also talks about the gaps between the reconstitution of the group and what he thinks of his patient and of the treatment. These gaps are a source of work for us and for the presenter.

The last member of the group to mention is the observer-reporter, who also remains silent, but from beginning to end. Their responsibility is to write a report focusing on their own inner movements and those of the group as they perceived, saw, and heard them, as well as pointing to the ways they may relate to the material presented. This report is the necessary support for the rest of our research.

In the next step of the research, two different groups work on the reports of the clinical groups that took place in the IPA and EPF Congress, the so-called Paris Group and the Reading Group. Some reports are studied in the Paris Group, others in the Reading group. The choice of which report is studied is determined by chronology.

The Paris Group, given this name because it traditionally meets in Paris, is composed today of sixteen IPA members who constitute all of the participants involved in the research. With some of its members coming from abroad, we choose to meet only one weekend twice a year. In order to be able to work on all reports systematically and in chronological order, eight members of the Paris Group meet half a day every two months. They constitute the so-called Reading Group. The minutes of the Reading Group meetings are sent to all members of the Paris Group.

To work on the reports in the Paris Group and the Reading Group, we use the same method as in the clinical groups; we suspend judgment and associate. If some of those present have participated in the group in question, they remain silent. Over the years, we have learned to read in the group work reported and in our research group at work on the report what we might understand through it: aspects of the transferences, the impact of the material and of the frame, and the relationship between the group dynamics in the clinical group meetings (and in the research group) and the sessions that were presented. We also gradually identified the processes that were found from one group to another and what the method used triggered, and have reflected on what this could help us to understand about the functioning of the analytical method.

We observed that the transferences and countertransferences of the initial analytic sessions tend to diffract on each of the participants in the clinical groups, each representing a facet of the analytic work. The reconstitution by the group of the analytic exchange, which often represents a large part of the patient's history and the history of treatment, is done by bringing together the various facets that were diffracted. We will say more about diffraction later.

We noticed and explored another phenomenon that is also played out in the clinical groups but which one could say is the opposite of diffraction. While by diffraction the aforementioned aspects are decondensed and differentiated, in this other phenomenon, they are concentrated to the extreme, that which sometimes resulted in explosive moments that can only be named as moments of transmission of sudden and surprising thoughts, and linked to the unconscious aspects of the initial material of the session.

We noticed also that the new treatment of the material by the research group (the first done by the writing of the sessions by the presenter, the second, by the group, finally, by the elaboration of the reporter) sometimes allows contents to appear that had been ignored or scotomized by the analyst, the group, or the observer-reporter:

The reading by the colleagues of the research group and the ensuing exchanges leads to further associations and we realize how much the starting material, that of the sessions presented, gives rise at each stage to new transformations, as if it was inexhaustible and therefore infinitely analyzable. This constitutes, moreover, what we have been able to identify as specific to analytical listening, itself also subject to repression, which can lift and bring up ignored representations during an interanalytic exchange, or even during an oral or written restitution of material. Even more specific, appeared to us what can sometimes occur at this step of our research (which is the work of the reports in the research group), namely the highlighting of what may have escaped the observer-reporter or the moderators or even all the participants in a group (Dorey, in press).

During the work on the reports, we questioned the specificity of analytic listening and the conditions that make this type of listening possible. The clinical material reveals the great variety of the analyst's modes of intervention, the handling of the transference, its interpretation, the interpretation of resistances, the relationship between interpretation and construction, and the work of dream material. Equal suspense, listening to all material with equal value, suspension of judgment, and attention to the effect of the transference on one's own psyche are uniformly required for analysts, whatever their theoretical orientation.

However, it appears, both in the daily practice of each analyst and in our clinical groups, that we do not always stick to these requirements. Resistance to allowing ourselves to be penetrated by clinical material and to surrender to the method of free association manifests itself in our groups in different ways; for example, by criticizing the method, the dispositive modus, or by adopting a supervisory attitude, sometimes by focusing on elements of the social and cultural reality of the country in which the analysis took place. This was particularly evident in a group where a German colleague was questioned about "the impossibility of doing a real analysis" within a cultural context in which the analyst must send several detailed reports to insurance companies for the latter to reimburse the analyst for a certain number of analytic sessions granted to the patient.

These manifestations may be related to the material presented, which turned out to be the case in the group engaging the treatment presented by the German presenter. These events also invite us to deepen our exploration of the theorization of the gap between theory and practice.

Clinical Material[2]

Two groups work on two different clinical presentations in adjoining rooms that open onto a wide corridor. From this corridor comes for more than half an hour the sound of a loudly speaking crowd, so loud that in each of the two rooms it becomes difficult to hear and work. One of the groups eventually interrupts its work by advancing by at least twenty minutes the scheduled break, while the other group continues until the official break time. The two groups incorporated this disruption into their exchanges and analyzed, separately of course, what had caused them to either interrupt or continue. If considerations of group dynamics were produced, they quickly appeared to us as defensive and related to a link with the material presented.

The report written afterwards (and the moderators *"après coup"*) describes the group that continued as laborious. The outside noise provokes movement, an act: a woman stands up to see what is happening. But the associative exchanges continue. This determination to continue comes against the risk of not being able to listen to one another in the group. This theme, not being able to listen to one another, was at the heart of the transferential material. The patient repeatedly declared that he did not understand his analyst's interpretations. This had already caused some noise and misunderstanding in the group during a session the previous day when the moderator reminded the group about the rule not to ask questions to the presenter of the clinical material. Some participants complained of not understanding this or that aspect of the patient's life and not being able to endure these misunderstandings called for the knowledge of the presenter – against the rule of silence to which the latter is bound. Out of this hubbub arose the fear that two parts of the group would not be able to hear one another. Those parts were supporting two different interpretative paths. Some of the participants thought that this incomprehension of which the patient complained manifested a feeling of depression, abandonment, dereliction, and sought in this complaint a melancholy core. The other part of the participants saw in this way of asking the analyst to repeat and/or clarify, a maneuver of seduction directly resulting from infantile sexuality, and considered this urgent repetition as the proof of an overflowing of the drives seeking rapid satisfaction. Here the issue is that of the loss of understanding; the external noise becomes the amplifier of the inner noise, amplifier by seduction of the infantile desire which would come to endanger, by its excess of excitement, both the work of the group and that of the analysis, which, in the fragment reported, always seemed on the verge of the absence of the patient, of the loss of sense, or the rupture between the patient and the analyst.

The group that interrupts the work is in a completely different dynamic. If the material provoked a brief astonishment, the associative regime quickly established itself in a rather large homogeneity which contained the rawness of the fantasies evoked in the sessions. It is a largely female group that welcomes the raw anxieties and fantasies of a pregnant patient, and the deep concerns of the analyst who brings the material about the future mother–child relationship. The group as container is even strong enough that a discordant voice at the end of the session of the first day can vigorously raise the question of the aggressiveness of this future mother against her fetus, which she considers an intruder. At the time of the disturbance, the group feels cramped in its "workroom," with the double meaning that it has in French (delivery room), and seems to have massively identified itself with the cramped child in a mother's womb that is too small. The material contained this detail of the extreme thinness of the patient which gave the feeling that her skin was stretched like that of a drum, enclosing the fetus. Identification and rationalization are an anticathexis (*Gegenbesetzung* is the Freudian term, *contre investissement* in French) of another series of fantasies, violent these, featuring a "serial killer." The material presented linked sexual fantasies of a repetitively murderous primal scene to infantile sexual theories about the "first grand problem in life: where do babies come from?," as Freud (1959/1908) explored in "The Sexual Theories of Children." The patient imagined the sexual relation between her parents as violent and painful, which is quite commonplace, but, in addition, dreamed of serial murder of women after sexual intercourse. The fantasies about baby making and giving birth repeatedly brought her back to very bloody and very noisy images of the cutting of bodies. Leaving the room, going to restore oneself psychically by going to see what was happening, allowed movement away from "hearing without understanding." Physiologically drinking a coffee and eating a croissant, stolen from the disruptors (refreshments from the other meeting's coffee break) was another way of restoration! These acts have been steps to enable the participants to represent the infantile sexual fantasies circulating in the group and coming from the clinical material, acts which, if we consider the psychic work to which they gave rise, have acquired the status of action-representation.

The isomorphism[3] between the functioning of these groups and their moderators and that of the patient and analyst thus became clear while, at the same time, reflected the difference in reaction to the disruptive event, namely the nature of the infantile sexual fantasies at the heart of the material, and which the group amplified: traumatic seduction in one case, primal scene and infantile sexual theories about the origin of children in the other.

It is interesting to note that a similar circumstance was treated quite differently in another working group in another place. This was the only Specificity group within a meeting of many other Working Parties. The atmosphere in this very small group was that which is often established within a minority in foreign, if not hostile territory. The clinical work was punctuated by moments of awful din: fighters on display were flying at very low altitudes – an air show outside the building. Although obviously embarrassed, none of the participants made any reference during the group sessions to this external event, which was not integrated into the group's material at that time. It was only in the writing of the report that the colleague in charge of this function was able to finely analyze this general deafness. The group, in order to maintain its cohesion, had opted for a dynamic that had taken precedence over the floating listening. This apparent deafness was also interpreted through the report as a particularly effective protection against the clinical material that involved a fantasy of child murder. Moreover, the SPTT Working Party was the most recently created, a newborn baby so to speak, and the environment was experienced as hostile and threatening to the survival of the newly born group.

This case of external noise may seem particularly far from research concerns about the specificity of psychoanalytical treatment today and may be a circumstantial detail. It is in these details, however, that the return of the repressed (that is repressed infantile sexual fantasies) is most likely to appear in a distorted and hybrid form. The hearing in the next room and the heard without understanding are infantile experiences of utmost importance, as they carry the unknown and uncanny, and provoke an efflorescence of fantasies that tries to address this lack. Whether a patient in analysis becomes concerned about the noises he hears in his analyst's house, or office building, or outside the consulting room door and tries to interpret their meaning or worries about the noises made by his analyst – those of crossing legs, intestinal borborygmi, sneezing, or any another, has always been in psychoanalysis understood as possessing meaning as great as the narration of events more particularly invested with affects. Such a shift of affects onto details, which in themselves have no interest, is one of the most well-known manifestations of the transference. And what is transferred comes from the original objects of love, the infantile sexuality.

The external noises had a different impact depending on the clinical material reported. In one case, the group that stops, the attention was focused on the pregnant patient, for whom the analyst was very concerned, as she feared that the birth, the arrival of the baby in the relationship between the couple, was an unbearable trauma. The group appropriated this countertransferential fantasy and put it into action: the third that appears and makes noise is a danger that prevents participants from understanding each other, and if they want to guarantee a future, they must move away from this disruptive third.

Here the child as an intruder and the noisy strangers are experienced as potentially destructive, while there, in the group that continues, the noise of the primal scene causes curiosity, annoyance, enactment, but no acting out. It can be integrated into the clinical material treated within the group, whose axis is the misunderstanding of seduction. The irruption of an unexpected event is often the source of fruitful progress in analytical work, if the intensity of the event is not too great and does not come too directly to reveal an unconscious fantasy.

The ear of analysts, like every human ear, hears more what seems true than what has been said. The analyst's personal analysis is supposed to familiarize him with his own organization of sexual fantasies, and how his listening can be distorted. His analytical training proposes to perfect her or his system of listening and interpretation, familiarizing one with his or her personal transferential distortions. But we know that there is not a training institute that resembles another, thus, the questions of training, curriculum, and teaching are those around which the most intense conflicts have developed. Such diversity should, logically, lead to very different listening. And, of course, this is what we see in international groups, at least if we remain at the most superficial level. For example, a French analyst will be more attentive to how language and its double meanings and ambiguities contain unconscious fantasies transferred in the field of analysis, while an American analyst will be more sensitive to the feelings perceptible in the patient and in himself during the session. If we stayed at this strictly individual level of listening, one would think that they did not hear the same clinical material and that their difference in education and analytic culture is so great that the specificity of the psychoanalytic revolution dissolved to the point that there would be several psychoanalyses. But if the attention shifts to the associativity level of the group, then the uniqueness of psychoanalysis reappears. The infantile sexual fantasies are diffracted in each individual listening and amplified by the movements of the group. The group can then be the place of the revelation of these infantile sexual fantasies and the psychic conflict that results. The group can also sometimes be the place of their repression as soon as they appear. Their identification is then possible only afterwards, thanks to the reporter's working through the material, or even by the Paris Group's reading of the report. These facts show that the "*après-coup*" or *Nachträglichkeit* holds a particularly important place in this whole process.

New Fields of Psychoanalytic Investigation

Numerous axes and questions have emerged during the course of our research in the clinical groups, the Paris Group, and the Reading Group. Some have been the subject of publications or oral presentations in conferences. Here we cannot go into more detail about all these axes and questions. They will be explored in more depth in our book that is in preparation. We use the group situation to examine the analytic method and how it works. We engaged in a great deal of questioning with regard to the function of moderators in our *dispositif*, the position of the reporter, and the way to work on reports.

Little by little, we identified and explored processes that are at work in most clinical groups and in our research group: those of replica, diffraction, weaving of thoughts, regression movements, acts,

and enactment. All these processes help to bring out the unconscious dynamic at work in the analysis presented. In the group situation, these processes are amplified. They seem to us at work also
in an individual treatment. Thinking about the group situation is a
complex exercise since the analytic processes are mobilized with all
their countertransferential dimensions. We have engaged in significant exploration of the group dimension.

Beginning with Freud's Wednesday Evening Meetings, analysts
have enjoyed a very long tradition of working in groups. But most
of the time, analysts do not take into account the impact of the
group setting. Kaës (1982) and Donnet (2005) have shown, in their
different but complementary work, that attention to the phenomena
that take place in a group promotes a better understanding of what
happens at an unconscious level in the presented treatment. We have
found the concepts they have developed very helpful to think about
what we were observing and experiencing. Other theoretical contributions have likewise enriched our understanding of our work,
such as the notion of parallel processes (Ekstein & Wallerstein, 1958;
Doehrman, 1976), and the notion of "field," introduced into psychoanalysis by Willy and Madeleine Baranger (1985), and recently
taken up by Antonino Ferro (2005).

Our groups are clinical exchange groups between analysts.
Different inter-analytic groups have been growing significantly over
the last twenty years. The modalities of these exchanges seem to us
to constitute not simply an organizational problem but a territory
of psychoanalysis itself, a new field of psychoanalytic investigation.
We believe that our research contributes to the clarification of this
territory.

The inter-clinical exchange group appeared to us as a space where
a certain number of problems that arise in psychoanalysis today can
be deployed and studied independently from any idea of supervision
and group dynamics. It is an area that already existed but whose
importance and interest as a laboratory has gradually emerged for
us. The inter-analytic group has become a laboratory, a place of
research and an object of research itself, in which the clinical material of psychoanalysis can reassert itself in its specificity, and other
facets of its specificity can be revealed.

In the group, the transferential elements are diffracted, i.e., there
are several transferential objects which unconsciously each participant takes on; several transferential configurations, and also several

components to each of these transferences. Let us take an example. In a group, a participant hears in the reported session the call of a little one in distress and wonders, "why does the analyst say nothing and leave him in a vacuum?" He/she is identified with the baby and conveys the reproaches of the latter. The question is taken up by the group, apparently as a technical conflict: "I work more actively," says the participant. "I would not do like that," confirms another. "It is quite appropriate," affirms another. One analyst says, "the analyst's formulation surprises me. She uses two negations. She takes the patient's formulations, does not say 'you,' there is no subject . . . she does not interpret." This irritates another participant: "I feel a tension . . . irritation . . . who cares about the analyst's formulation. I can feel her saying to the patient: 'your violence will not destroy us.' There is an enormous amount of violence." The presenter will tell us that he found in the group the violence of the conflict, which was played out in the transference, the hatred conveyed by the baby in distress, and the self-reproaches that the patient made to himself, as well as the internal conflict that the analyst herself lived in the cure. She is torn between, on the one hand, letting go and living with the patient, bearing the agony and hatred (of the little one) without understanding them, and enduring the undifferentiation, and on the other hand, the urgency of her own psychic survival and of that of the baby in the patient associated with a superego position, a cruel superego enjoining her to interpret, "because an analyst must interpret." The participants expressed one side and then the other of these positions of transference and countertransference, as well as the collision of these positions as if in a psychodrama, with these positions and their interactions represented and played out, and therefore made visible.

We can clearly see at work in this example the phenomenon that the Specificity research group observed and explored in its work on the different groups' reports and that we named, after Balint (1961) and Loch (1964), diffraction. The term diffraction is used to describe the phenomenon of decomposition that separates the different wavelengths of white light when it passes through a prism. Diffraction reveals the spectrum of different colors corresponding to the wavelengths or radiations that constitute light. In the same way, the prism of the group reveals the different constituents of transference and countertransference. Loch (1964) writes: "Just as the beam of light is . . . diffracted . . . by a prism, the comments of the group participants' break down/diffract the doctor–patient relationship into its motivating structure" (p. 281). The diffraction of transference elements does not involve lateral transferences, but rather modalities of the economy and topicality of the transference. These modalities appear more in a group, which permits awareness of the transference.

The participants are surprised to find that the group is very often able to reconstruct certain elements of the presented analysis, including an anticipatory element, i.e., foreseeing the continuation of the analysis, as the presenters may later confirm. This reconstruction can be understood by the fact that the participants, impregnated with the dynamic that is activated in the analysis, each identify themselves with conscious or unconscious parts of the patient or analyst and with their transferential-countertransferential exchanges. We know the dances of identification and counter-identification which play out in the dynamics of transference. The group situation multiplies them, and our *dispositif* allows us to identify them.

In our groups, we have seen that the whole group may be stimulated (in French: *être agi par*) unconsciously by the presented analytic situation and sometimes acts the situation out. Here is an example: one group complained about thirst, and the participants had the urge to drink water, tea, and coffee throughout their work before they were told that the patient presented was diabetic whose symptoms are known to include thirst, the need to drink very often.

In the group, each one associates through the spawning of their own thought and the associations of the others. The associative work of the others mobilizes unconscious resistance and connections in each person, which can in turn be taken up by the other participants. The associative pathways that have been closed or opened by one will be taken up by another. A double associative chain emerges: The first is that of the group, through the process of the unconscious elements that forces itself through and which finally delivers a story, such as the latent in a dream. At the same time, another associative chain issues forth, as participants observe that they find it difficult to associate in front of the others, but that nevertheless they associate by taking up something another has said, words that were not available to them before. In this sense, we conceive of the group as a place for an analytic game and challenge rather than just as a working group. Through the group's use of associativity and what emerges from it reappears the strength of this modality. We all know it, but like many participants in our clinical groups, we rediscover it each time.

Moderators as analysts are used to listening to the flow of associations. Here it is the associative flow of the group that they strive to understand and help to develop and unfold: what each person says, how the last speaker relates to what was said, and how the group constitutes its discourse. It is not to make the flow of associations a transcendent entity in relation to each person, but rather to see how this associative weaving in the group is constructed out of the flow of each participant's representations. In the written report, the reporter gives an account of the associative thread of the group and its resulting narrative. The work of the Paris Group and the Reading Group has shown that, generally speaking, this produces a discourse in which associations open pathways towards awareness of the latent elements of the narrative in the sessions reported by the presenter. Norman and Salomonsson (2005, p. 1284) give the group process the status of a "royal road" to understanding the material presented.

As a result of the different experiences of the Specificity groups that we have been able to analyze so far, it seems to us that work in the group brings an additional dimension of psychoanalytic reflection different from the work of the analytic pair, and that it also gives the participants a renewed experience of the strength of free association and its listening, specific to the analytic method.

Conclusion

Specificity as a Working Party has developed into a field of research that has evolved in different ways independently in Europe, Latin America, and North America. Each region has followed its own path. It would be interesting to further explore the similarities and differences, not with the aim to standardize our method, but to study how the different ways of working may have an influence on the findings. Beyond the differences, we share an interest in research on the analytic method, on the associations and processes triggered by acutely listening to it.

We have described in this section how in the European clinical groups of Specificity, and also in the Paris Group, we let ourselves be worked by, crossed by these processes, which has allowed us to describe them and to spot them, thus also to specify the pathways by which the treatment of the material allows the latent content to appear. What follows from these experiences in the Specificity groups and the work on the reports in the European research group is a reaffirmation of the strength of the analytic method and a renewed discovery of some of the processes which, through the use of the method, bring awareness to unconscious dynamics. It is also "like a glimpse of the interiority which is created in an analyst, which then inhabits it" (Dorey, in press). Diving into the experience of attentive listening to associativity and the process that this triggers is to dive into the experience of analysis, its method, and its specificity.

Acknowledgements and Final Remarks

The composition of the Paris Group has evolved over the years. Several colleagues have left, and others have joined. All of them have contributed to the research, and we thank them for that.

We have been organizing between three and five clinical groups for more than ten years, at least two pre-conferences per year (EPF every year, IPA every two years) with about a dozen participants in each group. It is easy to calculate that there have been several hundred colleagues with whom we have had the pleasure of working. We would like to thank them very much for their confidence in participating in our clinical groups, sometimes returning for several consecutive years. Their comments after the clinical groups were invaluable to us. We would also like to thank all the presenters who took the time to prepare the session materials, generously sharing their experience, questions, and knowledge. The reporters had an enormous amount of work to do in writing on the work of the clinical groups. Their reports constitute a very rich and always productive basis for the successive readings we have made of them.

With regard to the clinical material of the research meetings, we always pay great attention to confidentiality. This is a point that we insist on repeatedly with all participants when organizing clinical groups. In the use of clinical group materials, we have again ensured the utmost discretion in the use of the materials.

Translated by Jan Abram

Notes

1 In a previous article we have translated the French word *dispositif* by modus operandi. It could also be translated by device. We have decided here to leave the French word *dispositif*. In this chapter the term *dispositif* refers to the practical arrangements and procedures that are characteristic of the Specificity research group.
2 This clinical section is based on the article by Philippe Valon titled "La Sexualité Infantile Inconsciente: Son Appréhension dans les Groupes Cliniques de la Spécificity of Psychoanalytic Treatment Today" ["The Unconscious Infantile Sexuality: Its Apprehension in the Clinical Groups of the Spécificity of Psychoanalytic Treatment Today"].
3 We have used several terms in our research to name this phenomenon: replica, analogy, and isomorphy. Each tends to describe one aspect of what we observe whose underlying dynamic we are trying to understand.

Bibliography

Abram, J. (2014). Le miroir inter-analytique: Son rôle dans la reconnaissance des traumas trans-générationnels désavoués [The inter-analytic mirror: Its role in recognizing disavowed trauma]. *Revue française de psychanalyse*, *78* (2), 405–416.

Balint, M. (1963). *Psychotherapeutische Techniken in der Medizin [Psychotherapeutic techniques in medicine]*. Huber-Klett.

Baranger, W. (1985). La situación analítica como campo dinámico [The analytical situation as a dynamic field]. *Revista Uruguaya de Psicoanálisis*, *4* (1), 1961–1962.

Bleger, L. (2009, May). Diffractions [Paper presentation]. Association psychanalytique de France, Paris.

Centre National de la Recherche Scientifique. (2004). Spécificité. In Dictionnaire TLF (Trésor de la Langue Française). CD-ROM.

Doehrman, M. (1976). Parallel processes in supervision and psychotherapy. *Bulletin of the Menninger Clinic*, *40*, 9–104.

Donnet, J. (1995). *Le divan bien tempéré [The well-tempered couch]*. Presses Universitaires de France.

Donnet, J. (2005). *La situation analysante [The analysant situation]*. Presses Universitaires de France.

Donnet, J. (no date). *Histoire d'une recherche [History of a research] [Manuscript in preparation]*. Centre Jean Favreau, Paris.

Dorey, Y. (2010). *Libre synthèse [Free synthesis]*. Documents et débats 75, pp. 83–86.

Dorey, Y. (in press). *The Red Cover* [Manuscript submitted for publication].

Ekstein, R., & Wallerstein, R. (1958). *The teaching and learning of psychotherapy.* International University Press.

Ferro, A. (2005). Commentary [Peer commentary on "Field theory," by M. Baranger]. In S. Lewkowicz, & S. Flechner (Eds.), *Truth, reality and the psychoanalyst* (pp. 87–96). International Psychoanalytic Association.

Freud, S. (1959). The sexual theories of children. In J. Strachey (Ed. & Trans.), *The standard edition of the complete psychological works of Sigmund Freud* (Vol. 9, pp. 209–226). Hogarth Press. (Original work published 1908).

Freud, S. (1955). Two encyclopedia articles. In J. Strachey (Ed. & Trans.), *The standard edition of the complete psychological works of Sigmund Freud* (Vol. 18, pp. 235–259). Hogarth Press. (Original work published 1923).

Frisch, S., Séchaud, E., & Bleger, L. (2010). The specificity of psychoanalytic treatment today. *European Federation of Psychoanalysis: Bulletin, 64* (Supplement), 81–110.

Fonagy, P. (2002). Reflections on psychoanalytic research problems – A French-speaking view. In P. Fonagy (Ed.), *An open door review of outcome studies in psychoanalysis* (pp. 3–9). International Psychoanalytic Association.

Fonagy, P. (2004). Foreword. In P. Richardson, H. Kächele, & C. Renlund (Eds.), *Research on psychoanalytic psychotherapy with adults* (pp. XIX–XXVII). Karnac.

Green, A. (2007). Le pluralisme des sciences et la pensée psychanalytique, in La Recherche en psychanalyse Emmanuelli M. et Perron R. PUF, p. 28.

Kaës, R. (1982). Ce qui travaille dans les groupes [What works in the groups]. In D. Anzieu, A. Bejarano, R. Kaës, A. Missenard, & J. C. Ginoux (Eds.), *Le travail psychanalytique dans les groupes* (Vol. 2, pp. V–XV). Dunod.

Lalande, A. (1991). *Dictionnaire du vocabulaire technique et critique de la philosophie [Dictionary of the technical and critical vocabulary of philosophy].* Presses Universitaires de France.

Loch, W. (1972). Psychotherapeutische Behandlung psychosomatischer Erkrankungen [Psychotherapeutic treatment and psychosomatic pathologies]. In W. Loch (Ed.), *Zur Theorie, Technik und Therapie der Psychoanalyse* (pp. 269–282). Fischer.

Norman, J., & Salomonsson, B. (2005). "Weaving thoughts" A method for presenting and commenting psychoanalytic case material in a peer group. *Int. J. Psychoanal, 86,* 1281–1298.

Roussillon, R. (2007). Recherche et exploration en psychanalyse [Research and exploration in psychoanalysis]. In M. Emmanuelli, &

R. Perron (Eds.), *La recherche en psychanalyse* (pp. 103–126). Presses Universitaires de France.

Roussillon, R. (2008, November). L'Associativité et ses extensions [The associativity and beyond]. [Paper presentation]. Paris Psychoanalytical Society Colloquium, Paris.

Addendum

The North American SPTT is independent from the Latin American and European SPTT. Although certain facets of the work may differ, the collaboration within regions has been rich and fruitful.

There has been a close collaboration between the North American SPTT and the Paris Group. As a member of the Paris Group, the North American Chair participates in the elaboration of the method, study, and maintenance of the *dispositif* in North America. The clinical groups in North America share the methodology/*dispositif* with the Paris Group. The North American and some Paris Group moderators co-moderate groups. The North American moderators co-moderated with Paris Group moderators at the FEP and IPA in Europe, Latin America, Mexico City, and North America, and participated in the SPPT regional meetings in London. Further collaboration in the U.S. and Canada has occurred, with panel papers presented at the Canadian National Congress in Montreal and Vancouver, and at the APsaA conference in New York.

Analysts and candidates in North America are interested in the research component, as well as the opportunity to use free association and neutral listening in the group work, and have noted that they are re-reminded of the value of free association as the central tool of psychoanalysis.

Because English makes it possible to remove the gender references in the material, we have seen important reactions about the meaning of knowing and not knowing the body gender of the patient and about the way that this aspect may influence the work of the group and the diffraction of the material.

While candidates are excellent participants in the mixed groups, the success of the candidate-only groups in Latin America and interest among candidates in North America led to their formation in North America, in collaboration with the vice president of IPSO, who participated in the candidate group work in Warsaw. Work with Paris Group co-moderators in candidate-only groups at the FEP (Warsaw and Madrid) and at the APsaA conference with the Paris Group and North American co-moderators in candidate-only groups has been illuminating.

Notably, a paper by Margulies (2014) written after the first candidate-only group in the U.S. gives depth to the candidate experience. Margulies states,

> We saw that cross-cultural and cross institutional differences, notwithstanding, we shared more in common than otherwise. We experienced firsthand how our unconscious finds its way to the surface . . . blind spots became more visible . . . the candidate presenter felt less stuck after our sessions.
>
> (p. 5)

Further reflection among the regional groups about unique aspects of the both mixed and candidate-only groups is projected, exploring experiences in mixed vs. candidate-only groups, boundary issues, possible usefulness in training, experiences with free association and neutral listening, the uncanny, characteristics of the reports, après coup, the influence of the group work upon the presenters, and the international experience among candidates. Candidate-only groups possess some significantly different components from other groups that we hope to examine in the future.

The gap between theory and practice compels attention. Some believe that the gap is forever the place of the unconscious. Observation of the breaks (the interstices) between group sessions was discovered to be relevant. Use of the same methodology of the reporter/observer role in the groups was implemented. In New York and Prague, a silent reporter/observer who did not attend the group work or know the case material observed the co-moderators during the breaks the group took. Free associations of the reporter/observer listening to the co-moderators' discussion almost immediately elaborated the unconscious transference/countertransference of the case on which the group worked.

The unique opportunity to use free association and neutral listening in analytic group work deserves further study. Such study might include tackling questions like the following: how is analytic listening, free association, and the uncanny understood in different analytic cultures? The immersive and multi-cultural aspects of the work are often mentioned as valuable to colleagues from North America traveling for the first time both to the IPA Congress and to FEP meetings. They have expressed finding the group work of the SPTT to be a valuable anchor. The SPTT is seen as a vibrant, analytically immersive, international analytic experience in North America.

The work of the Australian co-moderator has made possible an association with the Pan Asian community of colleagues. He and a Paris Group moderator co-moderated a Working Party in Tokyo at the Asian IPA Congress (2018). Long-awaited further collaboration that was anticipated in Australia at the IPA Asia Pacific Congress in 2020 unfortunately had to be postponed.

Bibliography

Margulies, M. W. (2014). Out of the box and into the working parties: A journey well worth the risk. *Candidate Connection, 6* (2), 3–5.

4

THE COMPARATIVE CLINICAL METHODS WORKING PARTY – PASSION IN THE CONSULTING ROOM

Analysts' Approaches to Erotic Transferences

Marie G. Rudden and Abbot A. Bronstein

History and Methodology

The Comparative Clinical Methods (CCM) Working Party was formed in 2004 with the intention of "formally describing the types of working psychoanalytically." It was hoped that by carefully studying the actual work of analysts from different theoretical backgrounds that the differences and similarities in their approaches could be carefully articulated, compared, and understood. The WP developed a Two-Step method to this end, in which an analyst presents three or four sessions from one of his treatments to a group of 10 to 15 other analysts. A trained moderator leads a group discussion that lasts for approximately 12 hours; the time is divided over a two-day period. Each group begins with a brief description by the analyst of her patient and of the nature of the analysis thus far. The work of Step One (described later in this chapter) then proceeds. The group now focuses on every interpretation, prolonged silence, utterance, and/or behavior on the analyst's part from these sessions to consider what seemed to be the analyst's implicit or explicit intent. Six categories were developed for this discussion:

1. Did the analyst seem to be setting or upholding the frame for the treatment in the interaction?

DOI: 10.4324/9781032656311-4

2. Was he making a brief utterance, such as repeating an evocative word from the patient's dream, in order to stimulate unconscious associations/responses?
3. Was he attempting to clarify something that the patient said? Or trying to make the patient consciously aware of something?
4. Was he addressing a transference phantasy accessible within the patient's material?
5. Was he making an elaborated interpretation that brought together several threads (such as a transference phantasy, genetic material, revealing emotional relationships within the patient's current life)?
6. Was he saying or doing something that he realized departed from his usual method of practice (that which might indicate a potential enactment or countertransference response)?

After discussing these alternatives, the group then searches for patterns (Step Two) in the kinds of interventions typically made by the analyst in order to understand his underlying theories along five different dimensions:

1. The analyst's theory of psychopathology (what he seemed to see that was "wrong" with his analysand. For example, does he view the patient as having significant deficits? As responding to past trauma? As responding to intrapsychic conflict?)
2. His theory of listening (what he seemed to attend to, e.g., halts in the flow of associations, material that indicated affective intensity, dream material that illustrated underlying phantasies, hints about the transference as manifested within the given session, etc.)
3. His theory of therapeutic action (What does the analyst seem to think will be transformational in the treatment for his patient? For example, the development of a new kind of object relationship? The unearthing of deep-seated conflicts of which the patient had been unaware?)
4. His theory of technique (What does this analyst seem to think and do to further the treatment process?)
5. How the analyst seems to view the analytic situation itself (Is the analyst attempting to become a particular kind of object for the patient? Is the analyst focused on the intrapsychic field between himself and the analysand? Is he focused on the transference/countertransference?)

As the method has evolved, the different facets of Steps One and Two have been refined to inquire into many elements of analytic work as actually practiced in the consulting room. *At all times, the CCM method stresses that the group is neither offering supervision nor "siding" with or against the analyst's method; they are rather attempting to understand it as precisely and deeply as possible.* One aspect of this occurs through a comparison of the analyst's approach with other possible methods.

The Working Party itself consists of a group of trained moderators, a chair, and co-chair. All meet in Step Three to further dissect the material from the discussion groups. Each moderator presents the material from the group that he or she moderated, including the analyst's initial description of the patient and treatment, the presented sessions, and the group's work with Steps One and Two. This material always includes a description of the group's interactions, as these provide a strong hint into aspects of the presented material to which the group may be unconsciously reacting. These dynamics are also explicitly noted and explored within each discussion group as well. In Step Three, the Working Party delves further into the overall material without the pressure of the analyst's presence.

International Development of CCM Working Parties

Under the auspices of the European Psychoanalytic Federation, the Comparative Clinical Methods project was introduced to North America in 2009 and a short time later, to Latin America, supported by five-year IPA grants. Each region has developed and contributed to the method in different ways, often determined by the variety of analytic orientations within their regions. Although each region operates separately, we collaborate in the ongoing development of the method and its underlying intentions.

Prior to CCM's entry and involvement in North and Latin America, David Tuckett and nine analysts who pioneered and developed the method wrote and published *Psychoanalysis, Comparable and Incomparable*, a book that outlines the logic behind and evolution of the methodology used by the Comparative Clinical Methods Working Party (2008). Since this time, many papers have been written, presented, and/or published by WP members reflecting on different facets of comparison among the clinical models they have studied, using the data from over 100 clinical cases now amassed internationally.

In this chapter, we use our data to focus on analysts' varied approaches to erotic transferences and countertransferences. We initially chose this topic for a presentation at the IPA 2019 Meetings in London in which the organizing topic was "The Feminine." We had noticed after studying our cases that many analysts struggled with fully discerning and addressing erotic transferences in their patients. Further, we had noted that for women analysands, such material was often interpreted in the direction of unfulfilled dependent yearnings. After briefly reviewing the literature here, we will center on four analyses, two with female patient/male psychoanalyst pairs, one with a male analysand/female analyst, and a final female patient/female analyst pairing to exemplify what we have discerned in our sample.

Background

When a patient enters the psychoanalytic process, she has little conscious awareness that her treatment will evolve into a passionate connection. Nathan Kravis (2018) notes that among the many meanings borne by the use of the couch, an erotic one is clearly signaled from the start, at least unconsciously, to the analysand. Inevitably, hand in hand with resistances against this, or with use of the erotic transference to avoid other unconscious conflicts (Sterba, 1940), the analytic process will unfold with deep feeling. This engagement combines all the power of attachment love, the struggles for and against dependency, the longings to be seen and admired, and the fervor, jealousy, and rage that accompany erotic desire. In addition to tenderness, there will be mistranslations of intent, humiliation at feeling spurned or needy, punishment of the analyst for his neutrality, and an intense erotic desire for his or her love as an oedipal object. How an analyst approaches these passions is informed by his or her particular conflicts and emotional responses and will be shaped by his or her theories and method of working.

Ellen Pinsky (2017) comments gratefully on Freud's (1915) essay "Observations on Transference Love" for its provision of ethical precepts to the analyst to guide these passionate storms, noting the need for technical grounding in "confronting the immense power and necessary strangeness of the transference: that form of love, or attachment, a shield and – a volatile *something* – that fuels the process and can burst into flame" (p. 27). Pinsky notes that the "No" that sets the boundary against *action* on both patient's and analyst's parts in favor of understanding, along with the analyst's benevolent receptivity and lack of judgement, ground a process in which the analyst "performs as a deliberately incendiary human lure in a process focusing and magnifying the patient's love cravings" (p. 29).

Over time, analysts have learned to use their countertransferences, in addition to their abstinence and neutrality, to guide the process so that it helps, rather than harms, their patients (Racker, 1968; Jacobs, 1986, 1991; Gabbard, 1994). Attending to their countertransference helps analysts detect the disguised longings, phantasies, and feelings that are being simultaneously communicated and defended against by their patients, and to work with and understand their own reactions to them. The necessity of understanding projective identifications, which convey powerful, disowned aggressive, sadistic, and erotic wishes from analysand to analyst, and of discerning enactments that express subterranean unconscious elements of both the transference and the responsive countertransference, have further refined analysts' capacities to both understand and withstand the unleashed passions within the analytic dyad (Racker, 1957; Joseph, 1989; Ogden, 1979).

Nonetheless, defenses against a deep analytic understanding are inevitably experienced against the immersion in such forces – not only on the patient's but also on the analyst's part. To some extent, the implicit and explicit theories of the analyst may give shape to their particular form of defense. Some analysts may self-protectively react to and treat the erotic transference as something occurring "in effigy," that is, as a repetition of a phantasy stemming from the past subject to interpretation "away" from the dyad, rather than as something emerging from the patient that is alive and uniquely set in motion within the actual analytic encounter. Others, who strive to maintain themselves as stabilizing "good objects" for their patients, may distance themselves and their patients from the emerging material by using suggestion, educative interventions, or interpretations away from the points of affective intensity. Analysts who seek to "contain" what they see as material with the potential to disorganize their patient may inadvertently void the process of exploring the passionate thoughts and feelings that can emerge as aspects of an erotic transference. What we will demonstrate here is that analysts often do struggle with such transferences.

One reason for this struggle is indicated by Gabbard (1994), who notes, "Our psychoanalytic heritage has provided us with mixed messages regarding the appropriate analytic response to feelings of love in the patient and the analyst" (p. 385). Analysts are often unsure about how they can or should experience these powerful feelings.

Specifically addressing the range of erotic transference/countertransference experiences, Ethel Person (1985) argues, "Women in general appear to experience more intense and fully developed erotic transferences" (p. 166). She notes, from her consultations and supervisions, that "sometimes the tendency for the male analyst is to elicit but not analyze an erotic transference" (p. 167). A potential complication of this is that "one may see the perpetuation of a sexually toned transference–countertransference interaction . . . (which is) never fully analyzed" (p. 168). The impact on the patient is that she then maintains an over-idealization of the analyst, "often accepted at face value" (p. 168). Eventually, the transference itself may become a substitute for other gratifications, with a resulting "inability to mobilize effectively to form intimate relationships outside of the analytic situation" (p. 168) or to develop overidealized and somewhat submissive relationships going forward.

Harold Blum (1994) stresses the fact that "[t]he patient's experience of the analyst's countertransference is a reality within the analytic situation. The countertransference may not be just the fantasy of the analyst, but an actual set of responses on the part of the analyst, which the patient registers and to which he or she reacts" (p. 626). Blum goes on to observe that "sometimes both analytic partners have regressive reactions to frustrated transference love and to oedipal and pre-oedipal disappointment" (p. 626).

In the cases that follow, we will examine the particular ways in which psychoanalysts can react to the inevitable erotic transferences which occur in their patients. The CCM method is a powerful tool for the close description and careful understanding of how psychoanalysts actually work and why. Studied in this way, the cases show how challenging it can be to work with such transferences. We observe this struggle, as did some members of the clinical discussion groups who listened to this material, in a tendency by the analysts to use suggestion or to not fully listen for the signs of an active erotic transference-countertransference. We further observe a tendency to interpret dependency in female analysands rather than to address other contributing determinants.

Case One

"Angela" is a woman who has been in treatment with a male analyst over a lengthy period of time. He notes her history of unsatisfactory, even frankly abusive, heterosexual relationships prior to her current involvement with a partner who engages in "swinging" sexual relationships. The analyst reported a confusing and disturbing history of sexual abuse involving touching from an uncle during her childhood. The patient herself described this relationship as affectionate, while "knowing" it was, from an intellectual viewpoint only, likely problematic and "abusive" for her. Angela was described as portraying her father as either uninvolved or as critical during her childhood, but as primarily blaming her angry, emotionally inaccessible, "preoccupied mother" for the disruptive yearnings for intense connection that characterized her current relationships.

The analyst described the difficulty Angela had in finding words for her distress and her frantic fear of being alone as central to his recommendation of analysis after their initial consultation. He emphasized in his presentation of the current sessions that he saw Angela's profound sense of emptiness and loss as her primary difficulty, due to the disinterested or self-absorbed objects in her life both past and present. In his view, Angela's excitement over her swinging sexual relationship largely reflected a defense against her lifelong sense of emptiness. It was noteworthy, however, that Angela slept with her parents until age 6, and in her current analytic sessions, described feeling that she was her father's favorite, as he often sneaked bananas to her, which he did not to her siblings. The analyst did describe oedipal conflicts and overstimulation as additionally contributing to Angela's overall conflicts.

Throughout the sessions presented in the CCM workshop, the analyst and patient are discussing a trip that Angela is about to make, which will cause a long break in the analysis. She is travelling far away for an extended workshop. Angela introduces the idea of this trip in the first presented session after engaging

96

flirtatiously with her analyst about some common interests they share.

ANGELA: "I feel like a hamster on a wheel. Maybe I should take six months off, solitude. It would be nice to get up every day and not go to work."
ANALYST: "Or come here."
ANGELA (JOKING): "You could come with me! No, that wouldn't work. But it would be nice if you could."

She goes on to immediately relate her consternation about her boy-friend's saying that he did not want a deeper relationship with her.

ANALYST: "I think you are having difficulty talking about how you would like to find someone in your life who you can feel close to like you feel with me."
ANGELA: "I do feel close to you . . . but I don't really know you . . . I have constructed you in different ways over the years. In the beginning, I thought you were gay, to make me feel safe. . . . More recently, to think that you could be more in my life, my husband – if I had met you originally beyond these walls . . . but that is only a projection, me making you the good father, the good teacher. But it may be because I am lying down, that it is . . . all in my mind."

Later, Angela describes a power struggle, a pressure that she feels about his sitting behind her.

ANALYST: "I am not sure what the pressure is about, other than feeling vulnerable or frightened that I . . . will hurt you, or you will hurt yourself somehow as you struggle letting me get to know you more deeply."
ANGELA (A BIT FURTHER ON IN THE SESSION): "My intensity and passion intimidate and scare others . . ."

She then hears the next patient entering the waiting room and says that she does not like hearing this. Later that same afternoon, she calls her analyst frantically, saying that she had lost his cell phone number but finally found it. When he called back, she said, "I found you!"

In the next session, Angela relates a dream in which her former, abusive husband is coming after her and another woman and will kill them. Her analyst points out her recent attempts at dating, but her being terrified that she will be hurt, and guesses that in the dream she was attempting to protect herself from a dangerous situation. Angela speaks of the appeal of dangerous men and her "radical loyalty" to them.

ANALYST: "In the past, you have shared that you are 'analytically' in love with me. Perhaps you are struggling with the feeling that you can't be loyal to me while also looking for a partner in life. You might lose me and be hurt. You feel trapped."

Angela mentions how she understands herself much better now through her analysis, makes more rational decisions about the men she chooses. "But it does not make my life better. . . . It's like being in a cave with the best wine bottles ever and with liver cancer." She then adds sadly, "This has to do with my dad (who died when she was 14 – this had not been mentioned by the analyst previously). I had a special relationship with him." She describes him sharing bananas and other things with her as a secret from her siblings. After his death, "I was so angry, needing to find older men to feel special."

ANALYST: "You felt so alone and abandoned when your dad died and you desperately wanted to replace him, to find him again."
ANGELA: "I didn't know until recently how much I have felt this way."

Her analyst returns to her being upset about hearing another patient come in: she was reminded that "I spend time with others." Angela denies this, and the analyst adds, "Especially for someone else who will get bananas from me, so to speak."

In the final session, Angela curls up on the couch, speaks about how tired she is, and "in a little girl's voice," asked the analyst to sing to her or tell her a story.

ANALYST: "You want me to be a loving, soothing father?"
ANGELA, SOFTLY: "Yes."
ANALYST: "On days like this, I feel a pull from you to comfort, cover you, and warm you, to be your blanket."
ANGELA: "What is wrong with that?"

An exchange ensues about her "pulling in" men who are unavailable, such as her husband, who had been married when they began an affair.

ANALYST: "I can be a lot of things for you here, but I can't be everything you want or need me to be, and when you experience this, I disappoint you and I am sure that hurts."

Angela immediately turns to describing a problem with a close friend, whom she has not been able to reach. She asks for advice about what to do, and the analyst says that he feels in a bind because he doesn't know what to tell her, but he knows she will feel frustrated and helpless if he doesn't give her advice, as if she doesn't matter enough to him. Angela then sits up defiantly, saying that whenever she asks for something she is left frustrated and then feels very alone.

In considering this analyst's method of working, the clinical group immediately discussed his approach to the erotic transference material. They felt divided about whether or not the analyst was attending enough to Angela's past trauma – the sexual abuse – as playing a part in her excitement about choosing "dangerous" or forbidden, "incestuous" sexual objects, including him. Some noted that while the analyst did seem at times to consider intrapsychic issues, for example oedipal-level conflicts within the erotic transference (e.g., in his comment about Angela's being upset at this "sharing the bananas" with his other patients), that mostly he tended to redirect this transference by an emphasis on her finding "a man of her own" to share her life with. One member observed how much he actively discouraged her interest in him by saying that he can't be everything she wants or needs him to be. Several members agreed, concerned that the analyst avoided an active exploration of Angela's complicated erotic desires within the transference, including her seductiveness and aggression, her sense of "pressure" from him sitting behind her within the transference. They observed that Angela responded with frustration ("being a hamster on a wheel") or with an uninterpreted regression to being "childlike" when this transference was not seriously explored. Another member noted that the analyst did not seem to connect the dream in which she was dangerously pursued by a man with the events of the previous session, in which she had been flirtatious with the analyst, threatened to leave for six months because she felt like "a hamster on a treadmill" but jokingly invited him along, reacted angrily to hearing his next patient arrive, and finally called him very anxiously, afraid she had "lost him" via temporarily losing his number on her cell phone. The group felt that this anxiety was likely caused by both her flirtatiousness and her aggression within the session.

The analyst, who, in the last 45 minutes of a CCM clinical group, responds to the discussion, relaying that he felt strongly that given what he viewed as her past neglect and loss, Angela most needed him to be a stable, organizing object in her life and that a more active exploration of the erotic transference would have been "disorganizing." Some group members supported this idea, as they saw her as prone to destructive enactments, such as her sitting up abruptly, and perhaps, in displacement, making another dangerous object choice. Analysts often face this dilemma with analysands whom they see as action-prone and disorganized by intense emotions.

The Working Party group reviewed all this material as part of the Step Three process, as well as an additional fourth session offered by the analyst that was not presented to the clinical group due to time constraints. In that session, Angela described her boyfriend's anger and jealousy about her meeting with other men for lunch and about her not yet fully planned trip away for six months. While the analyst commented, "Somehow or other, I get the feeling that you find this exciting," he did not mention the excitement she seemed to derive from discussing this still largely unplanned trip with him. Instead, he suggested that were she to be away, she "would not have him in mind." It seemed to the Working Party members that this patient actually had her analyst very much in mind! We felt that this analyst's primary focus on Angela's dependency needs and on her search to fill an internal emptiness may have indicated an unconscious struggle against the kind of immersion involved in deeply exploring this patient's historically perverse and tumultuous sexuality. In fact, we noted that the name Angela, given to the patient by the analyst for the presentation, seems to describe a hovering spirit rather than an embodied woman.

The benefit of the CCM method is that through hearing many working analysts' carefully studied responses to his clinical material, the analyst may feel that his struggles with the work of the analysis are respected, considered, and offered for his reflection. In fact, we have often noted the struggles within analysts who are treating patients prone to action and to states of disorganization by their intense affects.

Case Two

Catherine, a woman in her 40s, presented for analysis because of emotional tumult she was experiencing during her first sexual relationship after a divorce. Catherine's history included a father whom she experienced as intrusively interested in, and critical of, her body, and who also regularly administered corporal punishment. Catherine had surgery in infancy that left a disfiguring scar about which she was quite sensitive., and she contrasted her feelings about her body with those of her female siblings, who seemed entirely comfortable with exhibiting theirs. Finally, Catherine's mother, whom she had experienced as frequently cold, verbally abusive, and undermining of her, died suddenly of a ruptured aneurysm when the patient was an early adolescent. According to the analyst, Catherine experienced this loss largely, at that time, as a relief.

When she presented for her analysis in the context of a new affair, Catherine seemed frightened by her accompanying excitement and by the fear that she might "lose herself" in it. She also reported feeling constantly flawed, ashamed, unattractive, guilty, and anxious. Before presenting his sessions, her analyst described her treatment, now in its termination phase, as one in which his patient had begun to experience deep satisfaction with a new, growing career, and an ability to tolerate a much wider range of affects, particularly with considerably diminished guilt and shame. Once her termination date was set, this analyst described Catherine as beginning to playfully express fantasies about her analyst leaving his wife for her.

In the first session presented from this period, Catherine mentioned a dream in which she was naked, examined by two physicians who comment that she "looks good." As she began to realize the transference meaning of the dream, Catherine became quite embarrassed, then sad about this reaction. Why can't she ever stop feeling so ashamed about her body? The analyst counters her question by intervening that, in his view, the dream was actually a hopeful expression ("you look good") that arose from within her.

During their next meeting, Catherine describes a new dream in which she was now wearing revealing but sweaty workout clothes to her session. This time, her analyst comments, "You might as well, as in the other dream, be wearing nothing." Then, he adds, tacitly referring to her tendency to subvert her exhibitionistic longings, that "in the first dream, you look good, but in this one, not so much." Catherine quickly responded to his intervention by saying that "this conversation feels cruel to me."

In the next and final session presented, Catherine talked about her relief that the analyst had not given her the bill at the end of the previous session. She had been feeling very uncomfortable about his last comments and hadn't wanted to face him in order to receive it. She then spoke about being angry toward her mother, whom she remembered as expressing disapproval about a dress she'd once worn that was "too revealing." To this, her analyst responded, "You are afraid that if we discuss your sexuality here that things will change, that I won't feel like your safe place, the mother you never had." He went on to explicitly reassure Catherine that she could have sexual feelings toward him without their being dangerous or inviting intrusive reactions like her father's.

In thinking about the sessions in Step Two, various group members spoke about Catherine's history of significant trauma: the disfiguring childhood surgery, her father's physical punishments and intrusive focus on her body, and her mother's sudden death during her adolescence. They noted that her analyst, whose theory involves offering a "safe space" that will not be punishing, critical, or overstimulating, had obviously helped her a good deal. But several members were interested in the fact that it was only after a termination date was agreed upon that Catherine began to playfully engage with her analyst about her sexual fantasies of luring him away from his wife. They wondered whether she might have benefitted from a delayed termination to explore her erotic and exhibitionistic transference wishes, as well as her shame about these. One member noted that Catherine's fear of the analyst's perceived aggression was not explored, but that he instead responded to reassure her, to remind her about the boundaries in their relationship, and to describe himself as "a safe place," "the mother you never had." Overall, many group members, as well as the Working Party group in Step Three, thought that the analyst's stance seemed to be one in which he was attempting to replace his patient's intrusive, sexually excited paternal figure with a "nonthreatening" external paternal object – even when, in the second session, she perceived him as sexually cruel. In the context of this overall model, he seemed particularly reluctant to explore the new erotic material during the termination period, but instead reassured his patient about the fact that her erotic desires will not affect the fact that he offers her "a safe place." He also attempts to replace a maternal object perceived by the analysand as cold and unprotective by becoming "the mother you never had." The analyst's theory thus seemed to be one that separated himself from becoming the hated, passionately loved, and desired object within the analytic process.

The analyst agreed with such an assessment as an accurate description of his method. It was the working group's feeling, however, that this model essentially foreclosed work that Catherine might have benefited from: the ability to further explore her shame about her erotic and exhibitionistic desires and about her unsettling phantasies about a sexual betrayal by the analyst in what seemed to her to have been a cruel comment involving her dream and her body. This might have helped Catherine to learn more about the phantasies connected to the inhibitions that she continued to experience in her relationships with men, as Ethel Person (1985) has described. In this case, the CCM method offered an opportunity to compare different theoretical models with regard to the specific dilemma of responding to erotic transference fantasies when one's model forecloses work on this within the transference, and when one envisions the female patient largely as having suffered from early traumatic relationships that need to be repaired.

Case Three*

Mark, a 28-year-old patient, had been in analysis for 18 months at the time of the CCM presentation by his female analyst. Mark was referred to treatment by his internist, when during a discussion of his erectile dysfunction he revealed in an offhanded manner having been sexually abused in childhood by his nanny. Mark comes from a wealthy, second generation immigrant family, has an independent business, and appears to be professionally successful. However, he realized shortly into his treatment that he does not disclose any private thoughts or feelings to anyone in his wide circle of friends and is always frightened of revealing his "crazy" anxieties. He is obsessed with sharks, watching videos of them attacking people, and is afraid of them surfacing even in his own swimming pool. He also is repulsed by messiness, feeling "invaded" by it and immediately, relentlessly, cleaning up. He had a close relationship with a woman for three years, but it ended; it was with her that his erectile dysfunction became an issue. Mark believes that this dysfunction is a punishment for his frequent masturbation since childhood.

Mark's father worked at home, yelling constantly, and was an abrasive, "invasive" presence. His mother has been involved for years with a group that follows a guru who claims to read minds; she believes that their prayers help many people from a distance. She is seen as superficially concerned but often emotionally unempathic, as when he told her only recently about the sexual abuse history. Mark's nanny began to suck his penis while caressing him at bedtime from the age of 7.

Some months into the analysis, Mark began to realize that his fear of sharks represented a problem with his own aggression. He gradually became involved with a new woman, who, however, was also seeing another man, someone Mark knows. In the first session presented, he described a dream:

> I am sleeping in my house; a woman is going around the sofa where I am sleeping. It was a scene in black and white, like photos from the '60s. I had a tremendous fear, thinking that it was my nanny. She was pulling my arm; I could not move. I woke up with my left arm numb.

A second dream followed when he returned to sleep. He was at a session, but at the analyst's house, not her office. Then the analyst became his trusted sister, saying, **"nobody is going to touch you."** The sister implied in the dream that she had known the analyst for a long time. The analyst then reappeared, and he wanted to know how she knew his sister, but she acted as if she could not say. The patient stated that he knew the sofa referred to the analyst's couch, and he was struck by the phrase, "nobody is going to touch you."

ANALYST: "You feel so frightened when you perceive that someone could get close to you, perhaps touch you."

The patient states quickly that he rejects the analyst's statement that he mistrusts her.

ANALYST: "I do know that there is a part of you that trusts me and it is that part that brings you here, but in your dreams the other side appears, the one that fears someone might harm you. In this case, it is me."

PATIENT: "Perhaps I just paper over the fear."

ANALYST: "Is it that perhaps all women get confused in your mind: the mother, the nanny, your sister, and any other woman who gets close to you? You don't know if I am a demon that may hurt you (referring to an earlier association of his) or someone to take care of you."

Again, in a dream just before the next session, the patient imagines his sister, the analyst, and himself walking together. His sister suggests that the analyst hypnotize him. The analyst tells him in the dream that he would lie prone between two chairs to be hypnotized. Mark then describes an embarrassing episode that occurred over the weekend, during which he was with a party of several friends, all driving drunk, one of whose cars got stuck crossing a river. He tried, in a manic-sounding way, to organize a rescue, feeling he could do anything, "like a superman." The authorities came rather quickly, however, and managed the situation. He then felt embarrassed and ashamed about his ineffective actions.

ANALYST: "Perhaps it is like you feel here, the current is dragging you and the water getting inside, and no one is doing anything."

After this interpretation, Mark confides that he was screaming during the episode, intoxicated, "I am the rescuer!" He is extremely ashamed. His analyst then says, "You wanted so much to be the rescuer, but then when you feel vulnerable and alone, there is a part of you that is very severe and even cruel with yourself."

In the final session, Mark reports dreams about toilets and about meeting the analyst outside before their session, about the analyst's toilet being dirty and the analyst expecting him to sit on something resembling a disguised toilet. The analyst responds, "In your dream lots of boundaries are crossed: private, public, your session here with me. . . . It seems you also have the feeling of being soiled."

This analyst, like many who have presented in the CCM groups, is using the language of touching, closeness, and intimacy to capture the way the patient interacts and responds to her and to his internal "objects." In contrast with the analysts presented so far, however, she spoke in the discussion group about her acute awareness of the various determinants of his sexualized transference. While she felt that it was "too early" in the analysis of a traumatized and paranoid young man to interpret these elements directly, she anticipated addressing them more directly as the analytic process developed further. She does, however, tie Mark's dream statement, "No one is going to touch you," to his fears about her, and she directly notes in Session Three that Mark is concerned about boundaries being crossed, including with her.

Many participants in the group discussion admired this analyst's broaching a traumatized patient's fear of her, and noted her putting his concerns about being soiled and about boundaries being crossed within the erotic transference into words. Within the Working Party group, one member felt particularly strongly that the avoidance of more probing exploration at this point in the analysis might be depriving the patient of relief from the pressure of this exciting yet terrifying transference.

Again, the CCM method offered an opportunity to explore the struggles that analysts may face with sexually traumatized patients who are experiencing an erotic transference. It is of note that this analyst did not regard her patient's transference as related to early dependency needs that were now being sexualized.

Case Four

This case is of a woman analyst with a female patient, Elle, two years into an ongoing analysis. The session occurs before a break in the treatment. The analyst observes her patient's avoidance of her feelings about the break and her muted aggression within the session.

ANALYST: "You wish you could deny the realness of our relationship. The moment you feel close to me, you have to push me away hard, so that you don't feel scared and vulnerable."

PATIENT: "I hate it that I need you. I want you to help me out of this. I want you to tell me to go away. (Silence) Don't say anything. I want your help, but I am afraid that you'll give up and say, 'Off you go.'"

We can observe a number of elements in even such short vignettes. First, the language used consistently throughout this and the other sessions presented is that of closeness and intimacy, of the analyst's stress on her patient's defenses against the "realness of our relationship." Elle's potential feelings of passion, of longing but also of defended-against excitement, particularly sexual excitement within the maternal transference, do not seem to be considered or explored within this model.

Members of the group noticed that the analyst's method of furthering the treatment involved making suggestions at times that the patient face something that seemed painful and hence avoided or denied by the patient within their relationship. The patient accepted her analyst's stated wish that she discuss her ambivalence about dependency, need, and "closeness," thus giving tacit support to the analyst's theory. Feelings that might reflect a point of urgency involving passion and the wish for a recognition of erotic fantasies and longings were heard by the analyst as related to her patient's very real fear about needing the analyst within their relationship. Members of the group, and the analyst herself, were intrigued by a comment from one of the moderators that she seemed not to hear potential erotic elements within her patient's material.

The vignette illustrates a technical and theoretical dilemma: in focusing primarily on relationship issues, the analytic pair works on something valuable that plagues the patient in her life and that is connected to real difficulties she experiences with the analytic work. In fact, such an approach in this analysis seemed quite helpful for this patient. At the same time, however, it forecloses the recognition and exploration of the analysand's erotic passions as experienced within the transference relationship. The analyst, throughout the sessions presented, implies a recognition of the patient's desires but maintains a focus on her fear of intimacy and of dependency, and does not seem to connect the expressed desires to a potential phantasy involving infantile feminine sexuality.

Intimacy within the maternal transference relationship might create anxiety because of the intensity of awakened erotic longings or a confusion about sexually exciting ideas embedded within these desires. These would be defended against unless heard and noted by the analyst in some of the patient's material. This analyst acknowledged that she did not see potentially sexualized longings as present for her patient nor as part of her reactions to the analyst's vacations, and found the suggestion initially disturbing but eventually as quite useful. She reflected on countertransferences that inhibited her from exploring her patient's sexuality or her aggression more deeply and acknowledged that the model she was using worked against such types of interventions. It was stressed within the group, however, that the gains made by exploring the obstacles to this patient's attachment security and to her sense of an integrated self seemed considerable. In the context of this chapter, the authors, who co-moderated the clinical group, wish to emphasize the potential loss to the patient of an emphasis solely on her difficulties with "closeness" and about feared dependency wishes.

Discussion

Freud became aware early on in his work of the passions aroused within the transference relationship. He also became increasingly aware of the therapeutic usefulness of unearthing and interpreting the infantile phantasies embedded in these longings. Analysts currently use their theories of therapeutic action, their practice of neutrality and abstinence, and their recognition of countertransference experiences and of enactments to guide them through the intensity of passionate dyadic immersion.

Both patients and their analysts, however, will also unconsciously resist the pull of such intense engagements. This resistance occurs across theoretical orientations and is one of the reasons for analysts seeking ongoing supervision. Some theories of therapeutic action that have developed in response to new insights about technique or about different origins of psychopathology may stress the interpretation of transference and of infantile phantasy less than others. What concerns us here, however, is the potential use of such theories to buttress an analyst's resistance to becoming immersed in his patients' erotic passions and the countertransference feelings these may generate. We point particularly to examples of treatments in which women's erotic feelings and fantasies seem to be reduced to "troubles with intimacy" or to unresolved dependency needs due to cruel, neglectful, or emotionally absent parents.

In the case of the male analysand, while his analyst mentioned his difficulty with someone becoming "close," this was "closeness" of a different sort. While not directly stated, the analyst was referring to a deep fear of women connected with a molestation, and with other elements in his intrapsychic life. The tendency to see women's erotic lives as suffused with dependent longings may stem from preconceptions and prejudices about feminine sexuality. Interpretations about the avoidance of "closeness" rather than of erotic longings, or analysts' need to reassure female patients that they are safe when exploring their sexuality seem to be relatively unique to analyses of female patients. This may result in female analysands not fully receiving the benefit of thorough analytic work that engages all of the various dimensions of their desire.

Notes

★ This case was presented by a psychoanalyst who is not from North America in a CCM group moderated by a member of the North American Working Party.

Bibliography

Blum, H. P. (1973). The concept of the eroticized transference. *Journal of the American Psychoanalytic Association, 21*, 61–76.

Blum, H. P. (1994). Discussion of the erotic transference: Contemporary perspectives. *Psychoanalytic Inquiry, 14*, 622–635.

Freud, S. (1958). Observations on transference love. In J. Strachey (Ed. & Trans.), *The standard edition of the complete psychological works of Sigmund Freud* (Vol 12, pp. 157–171). Hogarth Press. (Original work published 1915).

Gabbard, G. (1994). Sexual excitement and countertransference love in the analyst. *Journal of the American Psychoanalytic Association, 42*, 385–403.

Jacobs, T. (1986). On countertransference enactments. *Journal of the American Psychoanalytic Association, 34*, 287–307.

Joseph, B. (1989). Psychic change and the and the psycho-analytic process. In M. Feldman, & E. B. Spilius (Eds.), *Psychic equilibrium and psychic pain: Selected papers of Betty Joseph* (pp. 192–202). Routledge Press.

Kravis, N. (2018). *On the couch: A repressed history of the analytic couch from Plato to Freud.* Yale University Press.

Ogden, T. (1979). On projective identification. *International Journal of Psychoanalysis, 60*, 357–373.

Person, E. (1985). The erotic transference in women and men: Differences and consequences. *American Academy of Psychoanalysis and Dynamic Psychiatry, 13*, 159–180.

Pinsky, E. (2017). *Death and fallibility in the psychoanalytic encounter: Mortal gifts.* Routledge.

Racker, H. (1968). *Transference and countertransference*. Butler & Tanner.
Sterba, R. (1940). The dynamics of the dissolution of the transference resistance. *Psychoanalytic Quarterly, 9*, 363–379.
Tuckett, D., et al. (2008). *Psychoanalysis comparable and incomparable: The evolution of a method to describe and compare psychoanalytic approaches.* Routledge.

5

WORKING PARTY ON INITIATING PSYCHOANALYSIS

Understanding the Research Method as Providing a Container for Developing Thinking

Nancy H. Wolf

The North American Working Party on Initiating Psychoanalysis (in the future designated as NAWPIP) employs a research method developed by the European Working Party on Initiating Psychoanalysis (EWPIP). This method was developed by the EWPIP to study "the specific dynamics of preliminary interviews, how psychoanalysts work with them and what it is in these dynamics that leads a potential patient to enter a full analysis (or not)," (Reith et al., 2018, p. 4). The method was not theory driven. Reith et al. (2018) in their book *Beginning Analysis*, write of the method, "It is a hypothesis generating study . . . not a hypothesis-testing study . . . based on clinical work discussed by practicing psychoanalysts, using their divergent psychoanalytic theoretical backgrounds as leverage for more precise, experience – near observation" (p. 4). The point of interest is to reach conclusions about what in these first consultations allows for the creation of an ongoing clinical engagement either in a psychoanalysis or a psychoanalytic psychotherapy or what may preclude such engagement.

Through its research, the EWPIP came to realize that the work in the first sessions was not necessarily about lifting repressions but more often about bearing emotions that are not yet symbolized;

DOI: 10.4324/9781032656311-5

the EWPIP recognized that it made less sense to see the question of analyzability and the capacity to do psychoanalytic therapy as inherently residing in the individual and more sense to look at the analyst and consultee and see them as a couple needing to work together, both patient and analyst possibly feeling "at the brink of great possibilities and great danger" (Reith et al., 2018, p. 75). Reith et al. (2018) prefer to call this turbulence an "unconscious storm" because multiple levels of unconscious functioning are involved, and to distinguish it from the manifest emotional storm described in psychiatry (p. 76). The idea of an emotional storm occurring when two people meet is an idea Bion (1979) elaborates in his paper "Making the Best of a Bad Job." Both the EWPIP and the NAWPIP found his understanding illuminating to their research.

The understandings of the EWPIP were conveyed to the NAWPIP, and this knowledge provided a foundational understanding for the NAWPIP when we began in 2009. The NAWPIP continued to employ the European research methodology to study and understand first consultations. This method will be described in detail later in the chapter as will some of the revisions that were made by the NAWPIP. These revisions were the results of experiences the NAWPIP had in their workshops.

The particular outcome from the NAWPIP research that I will focus on in this chapter is the recognition that the Initiating Psychoanalysis method itself acts as an expanding container for processing the emotional tumult occurring in the initial consultations. This was an early recognition which with observation over time became both more evident and secure a finding. I will describe the process of containing as I understand Wilfred R. Bion's definition and description of the concept and process. It should be noted that the process of containing as an aspect of the WPIP method was not inherent to the development of the method but rather that this conclusion is an outcome of the research experience.

The NAWPIP was initially co-chaired by Ted Jacobs and me, and then chaired by me with Maxine Anderson and William Glover as members of the NAWPIP. Bernard Reith generously shared his knowledge of the EWPIP method and his experience as we got our sea legs. The deeply collaborative work done with Maxine Anderson and Bill Glover informs this chapter throughout.

Intent

In this chapter, I will share some of the work and findings of the NAWPIP to illustrate how the WPIP method can facilitate and provide containment. The chapter will show how the WPIP method in its containing provision, fostering reverie, offers the presenting clinician and the group participants a deepening emotional contact with and awareness of the meanings of the clinical material of the initial consultations. Instances where the clinical material strained the container and hindered the capacity for emotional growth and understanding will also be discussed.

The Concept and Action of Container/Contained

Wilfred R. Bion (1962/1984) develops the concept "container and contained" in his book *Learning from Experience*. In this book, Bion attempts to understand both what enables learning from experience and what prohibits it. He writes that the concept of container, when beneficial, serves as a model for a receptive and transformative experience that can facilitate being with an emotional experience for the acquisition of emotional growth. His model, container and contained, derives from his understanding the action of normal projective identification. Bion sees healthy projective identification as more than a defense, and rather as the primary mode of communication of an infant to his or her mother. Bion writes:

> Melanie Klein has described an aspect of projective identification concerned with the modification of infantile fears; the infant projects a part of its psyche, namely its bad feelings into a good breast. Thence in due course they are removed and re-introjected. During their sojourn in the good breast, they are felt to have been modified in such a way that the object that has been re-introjected has become tolerable to the infant's psyche.
>
> From the above theory, I shall abstract for use as a model the idea of container into which an object is projected and the object that can be projected . . . I shall designate by the term contained.
>
> (p. 90)

This sojourn to which Bion refers is the containing process, a process of bearing the intensity of the projection without feeling so

113

persecuted that persecution disrupts reverie. Reverie, according to Bion, is an aspect of alpha function wherein dreaming is possible so as to make sense and meaning of the projected/contained. The mother's reverie needs to be loving; if not loving, neither she nor the infant to whom she imparts her understanding will be able to bear or know more about the experience. If either the container or the contained is informed by envy or hate rather than love, emotional growth is attacked and will fail.

Bion assumes that learning and growth come from bearing the emotions, and tolerating the internal disturbance they cause. When the person containing can bear the impact of the emotional projection without experiencing the distress as an attack, it is possible to begin to reach a different kind of knowing. It is this process of being with the disturbance and holding in mind and dreaming upon that comprises the process of beneficial containing which can result in emotional growth. The process of containing is, as Bion describes, an early and necessary provision for emotional growth. This containing process remains essential for future growth and learning ongoingly; in maturity the containment may be an internal process, not always dependent on an external partner.

As mentioned earlier, both the European and North American WPIP found that the consulting analyst in the initial meetings is negotiating an emotional storm and that an essential task of the analyst in these first meetings is to bear the turbulence of this storm caused by the confluence of unconscious demands, projected anxieties, and transferences. This finding of the WPIPs indicates that the consulting analyst is in the position of container to the consulting patient's contained. The psychoanalyst in the initial meetings is negotiating the strains of the contained with limited knowledge of this particular individual's psychic terrain. The consulting analyst needs to bear the tumult without too much acting out or shutting down and hopefully with enough psychic and emotional space to find and shape meaning for the patient's communications. If meaning can be given to the emotional communications, thought rather than evacuation of affect can occur.

WPIP Method

The NAWPIP has recognized that the methodology of the WPIP in its inclusion of multiple looks and considered and attentive revisits to the clinical material of the initial meetings along with its approach to the material provides a powerful container/contained arrangement. The method and approach provide a structure and open space for reverie and dreaming over time. Bion (1988) suggests that the work of containing requires bearing uncertainty and doubts without experiencing these elements as persecutory. He writes in *Attention and Interpretation* that the analyst needs to pass through "patience," a variant of the paranoid schizoid position without persecution and arrive at "security," a variant of the depressive position before making an interpretation (p. 123). These states of mind are relevant for reaching understanding. The WPIP method provides such an opportunity for steady containment and growth.

In brief, the WPIP method consists of three independent views which take place over time.

The First View

The first view consists of the initial consultation meetings between consulting analyst and potential patient. The consulting analyst brings this material to the WPIP workshop through his or her process notes. The WPIP has found that the clinical experience of the consulting analyst is shared in more than written material, that the analyst communicates in words what is consciously known, and conveys and communicates other elements and disturbances through affect and gaps in knowing and sudden recollections. Since the analyst has been psychically holding aspects of the consultation experience in residues from listening and experiencing, and in dreams, night dreams and reveries, the responses of the group may unlock what is psychically or somatically held and provide understandings that will help for elaboration, remembering, and developing meaning.

The Second View

In the second view, the presenter brings the process notes from the first consultations to a clinical workshop. The workshop takes place for four hours with a break for lunch after two. Prior to the workshop, participants are emailed guidelines for the day's work and asked to bring them to the workshop. These guidelines are in the appendices to this chapter. Usually, the presenter's notes are from two or three initial consulting meetings. The presenter reads the process notes aloud to the group of 12 or so individuals participating in the day workshop. The participants receive copies of the process notes from which to read as they listen. These are returned at the end of the workshop.

In the first two hours of the workshop, the group members respond to shared process notes with their thoughts and associations. After listening to the analyst read the first interview, the group begins to associate to the material. After each read session, the group has the opportunity to speak and think. The participants are asked to connect their associations to specific instances in the clinical material presented. They are also requested to direct their thoughts or questions to the group as a whole and not the presenter. This request that participants speak to the group is meant to promote group dialogue and facilitate the development of a group mind. As we will discuss later, we have found, without conscious plan, that it also promotes the group's development of a containing function. The analyst is welcome to contribute to the discussion if he or she chooses.

We have found that the experience of the sessions presented, even if the consultation occurred several years earlier, has often remained emotionally alive for the presenter. This may say something about the case the presenter chooses and its particular meaning for the presenting analyst. Perhaps it also says something about how our psychoanalytic experience is emotionally stored in us as psychoanalysts. For the group participants, it means they have the opportunity to listen and respond to material still affectively charged.

It is a frequent observation in such workshops that the presenting analyst psychically holds and carries much from the original interviews, much that is not yet decoded or consciously known. If the group functions freely, not overrun by competitive forces, envy, or inhibitions, the members listen and are receptive to what is shared so that deepening perspectives are gleaned and can be articulated. The expanse of knowing is enlarged and deepened dimensionally in ways not possible for the consulting analyst sitting in the room with the patient in the midst and in the beginning of hearing the patient's story. When interferences in the group functioning occur, the facilitators comment on them or offer thoughts as to the meaning of such interruptions in processing. Sometimes it is only in the third view that a deeper understanding of the meaning of the dys-function and its possible relationship to the emerging meanings can be formulated.

In the second two hours of the workshop, occurring after the lunch break, the group takes up the open-ended questions provided by the WPIP. The questions are meant to provide some direction; they frequently revisit some of what has been discussed earlier but now are in psychoanalytic categories such as unconscious phantasy or transference considerations. The group not infrequently reb-els some about what feels like a constriction; most often the work with the questions becomes a deepening and expansion of what was brought forth in the morning session.

Structured Questions in Second View

The European Working Party on Initiating Psychoanalysis devel-oped a series of questions to be used as guidelines for the group's thinking in the second half of the workshop. Those questions offer the group a detailed and thoughtful look and opportunity for elabo-ration of the morning work. The EWPIP questions, along with the adaptations made by our North American Working Party, are in the appendices of this chapter.

The NAWPIP, after holding some Working Party groups employing the insightful questions developed by the EWPIP, decided to add two questions. The NAWPIP added a question about the nature of the internal work of the analyst. This question was based on the NAWPIP's recognition of the emotional turbu-lence each consulting analyst faced and the distress some conveyed. We thought a question about the analyst's emotional experience was merited. The question asked the group to consider whether it felt the analyst had emotional space for reverie in the consultation or whether the analyst's internal work was more about survival. This question brought to the workshop and to the analyst a further opportunity to reflect on the analyst's experience in the "storm." The NAWPIP also added a question asking the group to reflect on its internal work during the day.

The NAWPIP removed the question asking, "what will be the outcome of this process?," the consultation. Part of the protocol for the WPIP is to ask that the presenting analyst not share with the group or the Working Party members the results of the consultation.

No one but the consulting analyst knows whether the consult led to a psychoanalysis or a psychotherapy or to no continuation in a psychanalytic treatment. This nondisclosure allows the group and the facilitators to be in the same position of not knowing as the consulting analyst. It allows the group members to be in the experience as it evolves.

The European WPIP asked that the group members toward the end of the workshop, after listening to and working with the process material, make an educated guess based on the clinical material and the discussion as to the outcome of the consultations. Many workshop participants were uncomfortable with this question which seemed to result in the participants feeling they should know. The NAWPIP took this discomfort under consideration and thought that this frequent reaction to this question was an indication that the presumption to know required a shift from a mode of thought of introspection and intuition to a more concrete mindset. We also recognized that this move to the concrete set up an expectation in the group members that they should know and resulted in competition, rather than thought, between participants as to whom knew most.

The NAWPIP removed the question and decided to ask the participants, before the presenting analyst spoke of the actual outcome, of their thoughts about what might have occurred. This change from what happened to what the possibilities were seemed to free the group. With this shift, we watched the group stay open to further dialogue as they spoke about how they saw the patient, what they thought he or she could tolerate in terms of intrapsychic exploration, frequency, use of the couch, intimacy, etc. In one workshop, there was discussion about whether there was a need to see the analyst's face, and ideas about early trauma and developmental failures in provision were discussed. We found that this shift allowed for continued thought.

Structured Questions as Part of the WPIP Frame and Indicative of a Firm Yet Flexible Container

These questions in the second half of the workshop offer a further structure to the group experience, one deeply rooted in psychoanalytic concepts. The five questions regarding unconscious dynamics, how these dynamics are worked with, the nature of the analyst's internal work and the patient's responses, and the workshop group's internal work seem to provide a frame and a flexible container.

Workshops where there was strong resistance to making use of the questions often indicated a flight from deepening the understanding of the clinical material. One way to think about this is in relation to the concept of the frame. The frame as concept and action allows patient and analyst to hold affective reactions in an intrapsychic or interpsychic space so they can be felt and interpreted upon. Another way to think about this resistance in the group to the afternoon questions is in relation to containment and as a repudiation of containment and its transformative provision. In one group, for example, several individuals protested saying that "we have been there already" and voicing their desire to skip the questions altogether. We the facilitators began to think we were being rigid in our holding to the use of the questions and were seduced from realizing that we were complying with a destructive impulse in the group regarding containment. An opportunity for containment and looking deeper was derailed. A further description and understanding of this failed containing will be discussed more thoroughly later in the chapter.

Bion (1962/1984) writes that the container needs

to remain integrated and yet lose rigidity. This is the foundation of a state of mind of an individual who can retain his knowledge and experience and yet be prepared to reconstrue past experiences in a manner that enables him to be receptive to a new idea.

(p. 93)

The WPIP questions used in the second part of the workshop seem to provide such integration by holding known analytic categories while offering an opportunity for open-ended exploration of the clinical material; these questions reference foundations of psychoanalytic thought and yet hold and simultaneously welcome within that structure reception of new understandings.

The Third View

The final view or third view occurs after the workshop when the Working Party members meet again (sometimes months later) to submit the initial process and the group work upon it to another round of reverie which seems to deepen the levels of understanding of this particular initial consult. This third view will be explored more thoroughly later in the chapter.

An Example of Containing by a Workshop

In illustrating the work of the workshops and the containing process, I begin first with a workshop in which the participants struggled with their disturbance about a patient's approach to the analyst to arrange a time for the first meetings. Many experienced the approach as a destructive attack on the frame and seemed to be almost angry at the analyst or the patient regarding this. In the group work, a new perspective was generated and a new level of thought with a new idea.

In this workshop, the analyst presented a case of a young man who made several phone calls to arrange a time for the first meeting; with each call, the man requested another time, more attuned to his schedule. The analyst accommodated to each. The analyst presented process material in which the patient spoke of a difficulty in a present relationship which the analyst heard as speaking to a more neurotic level of his personality; in the middle of the session, he revealed a disturbing trauma from childhood.

After listening to the material, the group began addressing the patient's approach to the analyst. Many had strong reactions to the patient's imposition on the analyst for a particular meeting time and reacted to his lateness even with that accommodation. Group dialogue centered on the patient's need to control the analyst, and, for those who saw it in this way, it was attributed to an aggressive and abusive need for control. Some connected it to the patient's experience of domination and abuse from the trauma and saw the patient as bringing that experience into the room though his regulation of the scheduled time. The presenting analyst reacted to this and said that she did not experience herself as being controlled or abused.

As the group members engaged around this disturbance, troubled by what felt to them as a failure in holding the frame, a group member reflected on her own late entry to the workshop in the morning. She had arrived about 10 minutes late, and we were already working together when she came.

At this point in the group discussion, she introduced her late arrival as a way to think about the patient. She thought her lateness might have expressed her fear of speaking in a language that was not her native tongue; she shared her worry about being inarticulate. Perhaps she was flagging something she might not have words for. This NAWPIP workshop was composed of individuals from different countries but was conducted in English. Her identification with the patient brought a different vertex for thinking into the room. After this participant spoke, the patient and analyst seemed to become less threatening to the group; it was as if the group had found a way to consider the patient's interiority and the traumatic elements he harbored with less disturbance and judgment.

Interestingly, the group did not take up the worry about not having language for representing and communicating but rather took up the concept of time itself and the recognitions of how it can become fractured after a traumatic experience. The group member's identification with the patient led to a shift in the tenor of the group experience, moving from an all-consuming feeling of an attacking patient to one of having more space for reflection which led to wondering about the patient's failure to achieve a sense of temporality and an internal rhythm in concordance with reality demands. From that vertex, the patient could be seen to be bringing in something of the early trauma in this disorganized response to external time.

In the context of container/contained, emotional growth had occurred. The group was able to tolerate the disturbance of the patient's behavior and to move to another understanding of its meaning. This idea held the recognition of the devastation trauma can cause to the mind, in particular, in its destruction to or stoppage of the experience of living in time. The group did not abandon the thought that something of the abuse was conveyed in the patient's initial approach to the analyst, but that idea was carried with less judgment and fear.

This change in the group attitude and receptiveness can be further understood in relation to Bion's (1979) idea of the storm which occurs in the meeting of another subjectivity or other subjectivities. He writes:

When two personalities meet, an emotional storm is created. If they make sufficient contact to be aware of each other, or even sufficient to be unaware of each other, an emotional state is produced by the conjunction of these two individuals and the resulting disturbance is hardly likely to be regarded as necessarily an improvement on the state of affairs had they not met at all.

(p. 321)

It is interesting to think that this group member held and shared an aspect of dread of a new encounter held by the patient as well as by the entire group. It may well be that when this dread could be voiced, it allowed the group dread of its encounter with one another to be less persecuting and less in need of eviction. The group exercised its containing function.

A Third View

In the third view, the members of the WPIP Working Party itself meet to once again consider the initial consultations between the analyst and the potential patient and to consider the group work done on these particular initial consultations. The NAWPIP spends time working together over a weekend, revisiting the work done by again reading aloud to one another the clinical process and also the group process which had been recorded and then transcribed. The Working Party is then once again immersed in the clinical material as understood and worked with by the consulting analyst and further digested and thought about by the members of the participating group.

This third view experience continues the deepening work of containing. In this third view experience, the WPIP members are at a remove in time and space from the turbulence of the consultation, yet the content or contained remains psychically present and available, held in mind in a dreaming space and further prompted by again revisiting the clinical material. The Working Party members now have the opportunity to more deeply experience, contain, and bring their reverie upon the already digested clinical material and share their associations and thoughts with one another. This third view provides time between the group meeting and time within the weekend for gestation and deepening of meaning. When the work goes well, there is continued emotional understanding and growth.

In one third view, we, Maxine Anderson, Bill Glover, and I, thought further about a group's response to a consulting analyst's recommendation to the patient. The analyst had told the consulting patient that the patient was suffering from survival guilt in relation to

122

her psychotic sibling and told the patient that she needed to address this guilt in order to not sacrifice her own life. The analyst also recommended that she see another analyst rather than herself, something not spoken of as a possibility until the end of the consult.

The participants of the workshop had struggled with how they felt and thought about these recommendations to the patient in the beginning consultation. Group members valued the analyst's understanding and her clarity yet had some concern about her communication of the understanding to the patient, wondering if it were premature and possibly constraining the natural evolution of the work. One group member expressed sadness about the sibling being psychically expelled before the patient could integrate this sibling as a split off part of her own psyche. The group was working well, holding the affective concern and disturbance without judgment, and this containing work allowed the analyst to become conscious of something of her own which she said had not been conscious to her before. She shared with the group that her relationship with her own sibling may have unconsciously informed her recommendations.

The group's concern opened something for the analyst and in turn brought something to our attention for our third view. The analyst's recognition of her own history and how it unconsciously informed her work helped us understand more about her decision to refer the patient to another analyst and perhaps some of her interventions. Her recognition also helped us take account of the depth of what we as analysts emotionally carry. In this particular case, we were able to think about the unbearable experience of having a sibling or close family member decline and how it often marks and shadows the other's ongoing-ness of being.

We allowed ourselves to become conscious of the shock and horror experienced when a phantasy becomes reality, when psychological catastrophe occurs before developmental hatred or rivalry is lived through so survival can alert the one who hates that his or her hatred is not in actuality lethal. We recognized how deeply the survivor can be scarred by an omnipotent belief and terror that his or her wishes were the cause of disaster that did occur. One of us, in our Working Party, recalled a poem by A. R. Ammons, whose brother died from eating peanuts, apparently under Ammons's watch, when Ammons was himself a child. Ammons writes of his loss in his magnificent autobiographical poem, "Easter Morning." He writes of how the loss inhabits him, knowing it in fragments. He writes how he forever carries this loss in his body as a "pregnancy," or a sensory holding of a child on his lap, and in the shock, still, of mental astonishment. He says it is a feeling of something registered in him of not becoming; in wait; and yet inevitably gone; neither fully absent nor fully present; a not yet; always there waiting to be. Sometimes the reader hears this as if Ammons bears in himself imagined states of being and perceiving belonging to his brother whose life was so abruptly cut off. In this poem, Ammons vividly captures how early catastrophe shocks us, haunts us, and becomes profoundly inscribed in our internal world.

This case, midway in our research investigations, became a fulcrum in our understandings of what the psychoanalyst and the patient carry in these initial consultations. This again confirmed for us what the European WPIP found, that is that the work of these first meetings is often less about lifting repressions in order to make what was unconscious, conscious, though that was present as well, but more often about bearing emotions not yet symbolized. We understood that these inchoate emotions could evoke memories and feelings of experiences consciously remembered, temporarily inaccessible, or never accessed in the consulting analyst's own life. We recognized the depth of emotional disturbance that we as psychoanalysts may encounter and need to encounter in doing this work and the difficult emotional task of the consulting dyad and of the analyst and analysand ongoing-ly.

Failed Containing

In another workshop experience, we were able to see how the container was stripped of its beneficial qualities and how the container itself became close to a replica of the analyst's experience. We learned how the WPIP method's provisions could be disrupted, in this case by a volatile and disguised element in the clinical material that the group could not bear to know. The container/contained provision embedded in the WPIP method, however, offered an opportunity in the third view, post the group work, for containing, reverie, reflection, and learning about the nature and meaning of the combustion.

In this instance, the NAWPIP held a workshop in which the presenter brought a case from several years in the past. She had brief process notes; the group felt and spoke of something missing in the material from the start. The group nonetheless tried to think

about what was absent, to feel themselves into the presented process and make sense of the concrete thought process of the patient.
Interestingly, the group members were very in sync in terms of their
perceptions and ideas about the patient. More often in our workshop experience, there are varied impressions shared, and the group
members' ideas are responsive and evolving, not twinned. In this
group, there was a similarity in understanding which seemed almost
repetitious, and though the comments had psychoanalytic understanding, they did not seem to grow or deepen.

Upon reflection, there seemed to be a kind of deadened atmosphere in the group interrupted by a moment of manic energy. The
manic aliveness was generated by a perverse punning, which when
commented on by the facilitators, then deflated with no evolution
into a deeper understanding of its meaning. Later in the workshop,
there was pressure from some in the group to change the format and
skip some of the structured questions, expressions perhaps of hopelessness about learning anything new. Bion (1962/1984) writes that when
container/contained are "conjoined or permeated by emotion . . . they
change in a manner usually described as growth. When disjoined or
denuded of emotion, they diminish in vitality, that is, approximate to
inanimate objects" (p. 90).

It is interesting to think further on how the containing function
in the group workshop gave way to action foreclosing reflection
and growth. Bion (1962/1984), when writing about − K, attacks on
knowing, notes that envy can defeat containment and additional
learning. His thinking here is that some quality or reaction, here
he names it envy, resides either in the infant needing containing or
in the container (breast/mother). This negative quality disables or
destroys the capacity for containment. It may also be that the erosion of the container, as seen in the manic spurt and in the pressure
to bypass some of the procedures, resulted in the emotional load
being too much for the mind, for the container, to bear. When
this erosion happens, the mother, according to Bion (1967/1984),
does not receive and tame the projected emotional distress, rather,
she returns it, contaminated by what has been unbearable, and the
infant receives it now as a "nameless dread" (p. 116).

In this workshop, it was discovered that the consulting patient
came to sessions with a concealed weapon. Since the patient would
not leave the weapon outside the consulting room, the analytic work
was ended. Because the methodology of the WPIP stipulates that

the outcome of the consultation not be revealed until the end of the group work, the group only learned of the weapon as the workshop neared its end, and thus there was an abbreviated time for consideration of this new information. The weapon remained in the group's mind as a concrete entity with no opportunity to think about what it might stand for. The surprising and, previously, disguised contained, the weapon, disturbed the container, leaving dread without transformation or containment. Participants left feeling disturbed and shocked.

Containment in the Third View

The NAWPIP members had an opportunity for a third view in which a containing process was once again possible and in which the group's near replication of the consulting analyst's surprise and distress could be further borne and understood. The unbearable emotional element in the analytic dyad felt to us to be that of terror. This terror was unbearable for the patient and was attempted to be induced in the analyst through the threat of violence.

The Working Party members recognized that the presence of a weapon conveys a very real murderous threat which cannot help but drastically impede thinking, and often, if not inevitably, gives way to the reign of the concrete for each in the analytic dyad. We too felt the impact of paralysis of thought, just as the group had in their repetitive associations. We wondered what might have evolved if we had allowed the punning to find its own resolution, whether flight would have turned into some kind of knowing, or if we, the facilitators, with more time and space could have given it some sense. We, the WPIP members, returned several times to the process, and in time, began to be able to think.

At a distance from the deadened group atmosphere and from the shock and aftershock, we were able to get closer to what we thought might be the patient's terror of an annihilating psychic collapse into the maternal object. We were able to see the gun as a search for a phallic element, a concrete one, to provide psychic structure. We wondered if this thinking could have shifted anything for the analyst or how the analyst's knowing might have impacted the patient or what it might have provided the group. For the first time, we wished for a longer meeting time for the workshop participants, even another day as some of the Working Parties have in their format.

We thought this wish indicated that the volatility of the workshop meeting was still alive in us, as it may have been in the presenting analyst, and perhaps, in the group as well.

The Process Is About Learning Not Knowing

The WPIP method and process as developed in the EWPIP was informed by the intent to create an opportunity for dialogue between those with different theoretical perspectives. In that light, there is no one theory that holds authority in the thinking process in the workshops. There is an assumption that all who participate, since all participants in the WPIP group workshop belong to Institutes or Societies accredited by the IPA, are grounded in psychoanalytic knowledge and technique. The presenting analyst's clinical material is listened to not for technique, theory, or competence, but in order to reach deeper meanings and understandings of what transpires in these first meetings. The moderator(s) of the workshop acts as a facilitator(s) so the group mind can grow, and understanding can emerge. No particular psychoanalytic theory is privileged, and no person in the Working Party holds authority in terms of thinking or knowing either in the workshop or in the work done together in the third view. The NAWPIP has come to see this openness of listening and thinking, albeit with the structure of the method and with psychoanalytic thinking as background, as exceedingly valuable for the evolution of dreaming and for the growth of thought.

Conclusion and Further Thoughts

The research method of the WPIP, with its attentive revisits to clinical material of initial consultations within the context of the group process and in the Working Party's subsequent reviews, provides time and space for bearing the emotional distresses of the initial sessions and for reverie, dreaming, and evolution of thinking about these emotional disturbances, and thus becomes an expansive container and containing process. This containing allows for a deepening of knowing of the clinical material. This research suggests something of how we as analysts process clinical material and deepen our own knowing of our patients and what they bring that may lie in the realm of the unconscious and of the not yet formed.

Learning and deepening emotional knowing becomes possible when emotional bearing can be borne, and reverie and dreaming can occur. As with Sigmund Freud's understanding of free association and how it can reveal what is repressed, so containing allows for reveries, and through them, a finding of what is not yet known. In this reverie space, one experiences sensations, images, and thoughts that come to awareness as if floating to the surface of the mind or emerging from a deep dark interior, almost as if they have spatial and body locations prior to their arrival. These emergences then become available for linkage and meaning making. Reverie in the containing process is the crucible wherein emotional recognition can grow, as opposed to splintering into action or dissociation. There are layers to our knowing, and emotional knowing occurs over time as the mind can bear the emotions entailed and the insight acquired. The WPIP research method is a method moored in this essential process providing containing so as to deepen emotional knowing.

Bibliography

Ammons, A. R. (2017). Easter Morning. *In The Complete Poems of A.R. Ammons* (Vol. 2, pp. 14–16). Norton. (Original work published 1981).

Bion, W. R. (1984a). A theory of thinking. In *Second thoughts: Selected papers on psycho-analysis* (pp. 110–119). Maresfield Reprints. (Original work published 1967).

Bion, W. R. (1984b). *Learning from experience.* Karnac. (Original work published 1962).

Bion, W. R. (1984c). *Second thoughts: Selected papers on psycho-analysis.* Maresfield Reprints.

Bion, W. R. (1988). *Attention and interpretation.* Karnac.

Bion, W. R. (1994). Making the best of a bad job. In W. R. Bion (Ed.), *Clinical seminars and other works* (pp. 321–331). Karnac. (Original work published 1979).

Bion, W. R. (1997). In F. Bion (Ed.), *Taming wild thoughts.* Karnac.

Grotstein, J. S. (1981). *Do I dare to disturb the universe? A memorial to W.R. Bion.* Karnac.

Luzuriaga, I. (2000). Thinking aloud about technique. In P. B. Talamo, F. Borgogno, & S. A. Merciai (Eds.), *W.R. Bion: Between past and future* (pp. 145–154). Karnac.

Reith, B., Lagerlof, S., Crick, P., Moller, M., & Skale, E. (Eds.). (2012). *Initiating psychoanalysis: Perspectives.* Routledge.

Reith, B., Moller, M., Boots, J., Crick, P., Gibeault, A., Jaffee, R., Langerlof, S., & Vermote, R. (2018). *Beginning analysis: On the processes of initiating psychoanalysis.* Routledge.

Tuckett, D., (2008). *Psychoanalysis comparable and incomparable: The evolution of a method to describe and compare psychoanalytic approaches.* Routledge.

Wolf, N. (2019). Thinking about reverie in Bion's theory of the mind. In P. Ellman, & K. Kleinman (Eds.), *The plumsock papers: Giving new analysts a voice* (pp. 111–132). IPBooks.

Appendix #1

EUROPEAN PSYCHOANALYTICAL FEDERATION

Working Party on Initiating Psychoanalysis (WPIP)
Guidelines for the WPIP Clinical Workshops
Phase II

Dear Colleague,

We thank you for your interest in the WPIP clinical workshops and we look forward to working with you on that occasion.

We ask you to please read the following guidelines before the workshop so as to be familiar with them. This will enable you to participate fully and make your workshop experience more enjoyable.

We recommend that you read this text again even if you have already taken part in previous WPIP workshops. The WPIP's study of preliminary interviews is an evolving project and modifications regularly need to be introduced. As a result, this text is different in places from earlier versions that you may have studied. In particular, Section 4 is a completely new version that was introduced for the workshops that were held at the 2009 EPF Conference in Brussels, and even there some changes have been introduced on the basis of the Brussels experience.

1. Introduction to the Workshop Method

The aim of the WPIP workshops is to investigate what happens in preliminary interviews that subsequently lead to successful psychoanalyses. Presumably, something is done that 1) allows the analyst to judge that the patient can benefit from full analysis (we may call this the "assessment" aspect of the interview) and 2) allows the patient to arrive at a personal conviction that it would indeed be worth his while to get this kind of treatment (the "motivation" aspect). In the long run, better understanding of this process should help us not only to improve our criteria for indicating psychoanalysis or for recommending another form of treatment, but also to get more analyses going with suitable patients as the result of more competently handled and motivating interviews.

The WPIP's present thinking on the issue is that the assessment and motivation aspects are probably closely linked. Both seem to require the analyst to set off or "initiate" some form of psychoanalytic process which allows him to judge how the patient responds to it and which simultaneously allows the patient to get a direct experience of what analysis is about and what it has to offer that is specific and valuable. Although there may be significant differences between the initiation process in "consultation" settings, where the interviewing analyst is evaluating the indication for referral to another analyst, and "private" settings, where the analysis will continue with the interviewing analyst, we presume that there will also be aspects of the process that are common to both settings and that allow the patient to get a "taste" of psychoanalysis.

The question then is how that "initial" psychoanalytic process works and how analyst and patient manage to "switch the level" from an ordinary kind of interview to a specifically psychoanalytic one. In order to avoid *a priori* definitions of what should be considered "specifically psychoanalytic," it may be worthwhile to take a fresh look at real clinical material in order to find out what it can tell us about competent contemporary psychoanalytic practice.

The general plan for the WPIP workshops is to ask experienced analysts to present transcripts of an initial interview, or series of such interviews, and to explore with the analyst what it is that experienced analysts actually do in such settings. The idea is that the analyst has not only explicit knowledge about what he does, and about which he can tell us directly, but also implicit knowledge that the group can help him to formulate or discover together with him. Through this collaboration with the presenting analyst, we may be able to detect patterns in the clinical material that strike us as potentially significant. We can then try to describe these patterns in ways that are both as simple as possible and as close as possible to clinical experience.

The comparison of such patterns across many cases may help us to reach a consensus about some commonly encountered characteristics of preliminary interviews and help us to improve our understanding of the interview process. This can only be done in a stepwise, recursive process in which very general ideas lead to observations that help us to refine our thinking, generating new ideas that in turn allow us to make more precise observations, and so on.

2. A New Step in the Research Project: The Workshops Will Be "Blind" to the Outcome of the Interviews

Previous WPIP workshops at the EPF Annual Conferences in Vilamoura (2005), Athens (2006), and Barcelona (2007), as well as at the IPA Conference in Berlin in July 2007, were designed to investigate the dynamics of preliminary interviews that led to successful psychoanalyses. Workshop participants knew from the outset that they would be studying interviews that led to full psychoanalysis. Their task therefore was not to predict the outcome, but rather to use the clinical material to try to detect and describe the interview dynamics that might help to make sense of the outcome. Some preliminary ideas have emerged from this material which we will not describe here, so as not to influence you, but which will be published in an upcoming issue of the EPF Bulletin.

A new phase in this project began with trial workshops held at the 2008 EPF Conference in Vienna. This phase has involved the WPIP is extending its study to include preliminary interviews that did *not* lead to psychoanalysis, resulting, for example, in psychotherapy or in no treatment at all. There are two main ideas behind this new phase: The first is that if the discussion is not influenced by certain knowledge of the outcome, it should be even more open and exploratory. The second is that extending the case material to interviews that did not necessarily lead to full psychoanalysis will allow us to look at a potentially greater variety of interview dynamics and explore possible relationships, if any, between these dynamics and outcome. Any differences, or their absence, would help us to refine our understanding of the process of initiating psychoanalysis.

The plan is thus to let the workshops begin by working "blind" to the results of the interviews. The presenters will bring material from a case that they found particularly interesting, but neither in their presentation nor in their written case material will they reveal anything about the outcome of the interviews, for example, what form of treatment they proposed to the patient or how the patient reacted to the recommendation. The workshops' twofold task will be to see if they can "predict" the outcome of the interviews, and to justify their predictions on the basis of the dynamics that they think they see at work in the case material. Participants will be informed about the actual outcome only towards the end of the workshops, where some time will be set aside to discuss the relationships between the workshop's prediction and the actual outcome.

3.   Practical Organization of the Workshops

The workshops will be held in two sessions of two hours each. The first session will be devoted to the case presentation, lasting 45 to 60 minutes, followed by a free discussion within the group and with the presenting analyst. Your participation in both sessions is of course essential.

In the second session this discussion will be pursued in a semi-structured manner, using four questions that you will be asked to answer on the basis of the material. The questions were developed on the basis of the Vienna experience and were applied successfully in the workshops at the EPF Conferences in Brussels (2009) and London (2010), as well as at the IPA Conference in Chicago in 2009.

In New York in 2011, after the second session, we will have some extra time to discuss the workshop process and experience as well.

4.   Questions for the Workshops

The very general questions that we ask you to keep in mind throughout the workshop proceedings are the following:

What do you think that this patient and this interviewing analyst decided that it would be worthwhile for the patient to do as a result of this (these) preliminary interview(s)? What do you think lies behind their decision(s), and how do you explain this on the basis of what you can see in the interview dynamics? Finally, what is the evidence for your inferences?

Our basic hypothesis in examining these cases is that the patient and analyst "know" what they are doing and that their decisions are well grounded, even if this "knowledge" may sometimes be unconscious or implicit. Remember that the patient and the analyst may arrive at different conclusions and that they may both have good reasons for this from within their own respective perspective. Our task is to find out how to describe the "ground" on which their decision(s) were made.

A corollary hypothesis is that a psychoanalytically meaningful process leading to valid treatment and/or referral options can take place in both "private" and "consultation" settings (see p. 1 for an explanation of this distinction). Our task is to try to describe what is fundamental about this process.

In order to give some structure to your examination of the case, we ask you to look at it from four related points of view embedded in the four questions asked below. If the workshops make sure to address all four questions, this will make it easier for the WPIP to compare the outcomes of different workshops.

The examples or explanations given under each question should not be seen as mandatory or comprehensive. They are only there to illustrate the kinds of things you may want to look for. You should feel free to answer the questions in your own way if you believe that this is called for by the material or by your own understanding of it.

However, in all cases we ask you to please cite your *evidence* for your observations (see also Section 6 below).

4.1 What Unconscious Dynamics Are at Work in This Encounter?

For example, what are the unconscious issues that the patient brings to the interview(s)? How are they related to expectations about help or treatment? What are the most important transference and countertransference dynamics that seem to be at work? How do they evolve? Is there a moment in the unconscious dynamics that you would consider to be very important for the development of the interview(s) and for the probable outcome? Could there be unconscious issues that are avoided? Does this seem to influence the outcome in one way or another? Please cite evidence for your hypotheses, in particular by referring to illustrative moments in the case material.

4.2 How Do We See the Analyst Working With These Dynamics?

The basic hypothesis is that the process being studied is the result of a specifically psychoanalytic encounter between this particular analyst and this particular patient. How do we see the analyst working to make this encounter possible? How does he work with the unconscious dynamics? What does he listen for, what is he attentive to? What is his general style of working? What does he say or not say that seems to be important? How is this related to his understanding of the patient? What kind of internal work does the analyst do and how does this influence his work with the patient? It will of course be important to check your hypotheses about how the analyst works by discussing them with the analyst.

4.3 How Do We See the Patient Responding to How the Analyst Works?

This question naturally refers both to the patient's overt, conscious responses and to what you think you can infer about the patient's unconscious processes. For example, what does this material reveal about the patient's intrapsychic functioning? What does it suggest about the patient's ability to use the analyst and/or the analytic setting? Can you see psychic movement in the patient's responses? How would you describe it? Alternatively, what does not change? Is the movement, if any, related to the psychoanalytic process, and how? Once again, we ask you to find evidence for your observations, based on the process material and your discussion of it with the analyst.

4.4 What Will Be the Outcome of This Process?

What do you think will happen after this (these) interview(s)? What will be this analyst's offer or recommendation to this patient? Psychoanalysis, psychoanalytic psychotherapy, or some other option? Why? How will the patient react to the offer, and what course of action will he follow? Why? What kind of process do you predict is likely to take place in the resulting treatment? How do you think that the patient will be able to benefit from it? What kinds of difficulties do you think are likely to be encountered? Please try to find evidence for your predictions in the material and then discuss it with the analyst once the outcome has been revealed.

5. Confidentiality

Work like this necessarily involves highly confidential and sensitive clinical material. It is feasible only if the utmost care is taken at all steps to protect the identity of the patients involved. Furthermore, given the personal involvement of the presenting analyst, as well as that of the other workshop participants, in a psychoanalytic group process, there must be a safe environment in which everyone can feel free to express his or her own thoughts.

For these reasons, all participants are expected to maintain total confidentiality outside the workshops about everything that took place inside, including, of course, the case material, but also the name of the presenter and opinions expressed by the participants.

To facilitate your participation in the workshop, the presenter will distribute written copies of his or her clinical material. This will also allow you to refer back to precise sequences in the material during the discussion. You are required to hand back your copy to the presenter personally before you leave the workshop.

With the permission of the presenting analyst, the workshop discussions are audio-recorded for later re-analysis by the WPIP. This and all other data will be handled with absolute confidentiality towards the patient, the presenter, and the workshop participants.

6. Other Recommendations

To help you to understand this approach, it may be useful to add some comments to explain the WPIP's thinking about where the information that we need is to be found, what the information can tell us, and what ways can best be used to describe it.

The WPIP suggests that in the group method proposed here, *the ultimate source of the data is the mind of the presenter.* The analyst presenting the case is the one who has the knowledge that we need about what happened during the interview being studied. He or she holds this knowledge in various forms: theories, fantasies, images, emotions stirred up by the patient, body sensations, and so on. Some of this knowledge will be explicit but some of it will be implicit and/or unconscious. The group's function is to help the presenter to bring this out and to give it meaning. Some of the information will be present in the written transcript; some of it will become apparent while the presenter reads this text; but still more will come forth only in the discussion. We want to insist here that the group's own fantasies and theories about the case do *not* constitute knowledge as such, and that there is little use in disputing directly about competing fantasies and models. These elements that inevitably arise in the group *are* useful however, if they are used as part of the exploration with the analyst because they may help the latter to say more about his or her explicit and implicit knowledge about the case.

This workshop procedure may work best if the workshop begins its examination of the case material without involving the presenting analyst directly, but of course it will be essential to discuss it periodically with him or her as just described, and then again once the workshop's predictions have been made and the true outcome has been revealed.

As to what the information can teach us, we suggest that when we analyze session transcripts, as well as the analyst's own impressions, what we are mainly seeing at this stage is *a text produced by the analytic couple*. Even though it may be tempting to dissect the material to isolate a "typical" patient or a "typical" analytic technique, we must recognize that our real ability to do this is rather limited when analyzing a few sessions from a single case. The session is the result of innumerable and often very subtle contributions from both patient and analyst, who are constantly interacting with each other in inextricable ways so that if we look carefully at what happens, we may find that we cannot confidently discern a particular kind of patient, nor a particular kind of analyst, but only a particular kind of relationship or interaction between the two of them, i.e., the creation of an analytic couple. Thus, for example, if we see shifts in the course of the interview, we might be seeing shifts not only in the mind of the patient, but also in the minds of both the patient and the analyst working together.

In this context, it is essential to remember that *the aim of this kind of work is to learn from the clinical material, not to judge it*. For example, one finding of this kind of research could be that *there may be several different ways of doing effective preliminary interviews.* These might "work" in different ways but they might all lead to good indications for analysis or for other forms of analytic treatment. The problem is then to try to discern *how* each approach works, not to emphasize or vindicate one's own preferred method or theory.

Finally, a word about *how best to describe observations drawn from clinical material.* Psychoanalytic terminology can be useful here, but it can also be an obstacle. One problem is that our psychoanalytic concepts can lead us to search the material only for what they lead us to expect, thus preventing us from taking a fresh look and making new observations. Another problem is that the relationships between psychoanalytic terms, the concepts they refer to, and finally the observations that those concepts are meant to describe, has become extremely complex. The same term can have rather different meanings in different psychoanalytic cultures, and apparently unrelated concepts can be used to refer to very similar phenomena. Even within a given school of analytic thinking, individual analysts may use the same explicit terminology to refer to rather different implicit personal theories. One helpful way to avoid the misunderstandings that can arise from these differences is to use the actual clinical material to illustrate what one is trying to say. Another way may be to take one step backwards from our usual terminology and to begin by using ordinary language to describe possible patterns in the material. This may provide the extra mental space we need for a renewed, playful, and creative interaction between our psychoanalytic concepts and the clinical data. Once a consensus has been reached about an observation, we can always try to translate it back into existing psychoanalytic terminology, if appropriate.

This means that it will be important to *illustrate all observations, descriptions, and conclusions with specific examples drawn from the case material,* such as sequences in the patient–analyst interaction that seem significant, shifts in the contents of the patient's fantasies that are interesting or unexpected, interpretations or other interventions that look particularly effective, etc. These illustrative examples will help to ground the workshop's observations and conclusions. They will also provide precious data for further elaboration by the WPIP. For example, if two workshops use similar language to describe significant patterns that they have discerned in the case material, it is impossible to tell whether these descriptions actually correspond to comparable phenomena unless they are accompanied by specific illustrations.

This is an ongoing conceptual and participative research effort which is designed to change as it progresses. Your feedback concerning the procedure and your workshop experiences will be highly appreciated and will help the WPIP to make improvements.

My WPIP colleagues and I thank you very much for your contribution, and we hope that you will find the whole experience useful and stimulating!

Bernard Reith for the WPIP
January 2011

NORTH AMERICAN WORKING PARTY ON INITIATING PSYCHOANALYSIS (WPIP)

Guidelines for WPIP clinical workshops (6.20.13)
(Adapted from the guidelines of the European Psychoanalytic Federation WPIP)

★ This appendix contains the NAWPIP changes made to the EWPIP Guidelines.

NOTE: The North American WPIP workshops will continue to begin "blind" to the outcome of the interviews, but we will hold off on predicting the outcome. The Working Party feels this will maintain an open, exploratory discussion. Other than the presenter, no one will know if the consultation led to analysis or not, and the presenter will not disclose his recommendation or the patient's response until the conclusion of the workshop. The workshop questions in Section 4 have been altered accordingly.

4. Questions for the workshops (**Here are included all the questions for the Workshops. The additional questions of the NAWPIP are in bold and with the names of the NAWPIP Working Party**)

The very general questions that we ask you to keep in mind throughout the workshop proceedings are the following:

4.1 What Unconscious Dynamics Are at Work in This Encounter?

For example, what are the unconscious issues that the patient brings to the interview(s)? How are they related to expectations about help or treatment? What are the most important transference and countertransference dynamics that seem to be at work? How do they evolve? Is there a moment in the unconscious dynamics that you would consider to be very important for the development of the interview(s) and for the probable outcome? Could there be unconscious issues that are avoided? Does this seem to influence the outcome in one way or another? Please cite evidence for your hypotheses by referring to illustrative moments in the case material.

4.2   How Do We See the Analyst Working With These Dynamics?

The basic hypothesis is that the process being studied is the result of a specifically psychoanalytic encounter between this particular analyst and this particular patient. How do we see the analyst working to make this encounter possible? How does he work with the unconscious dynamics? What does he listen for, what is he attentive to? What is his general style of working? What does he say or not say that seems to be important? How is this related to his understanding of the patient? Again, please cite evidence in the text.

4.3   What Is the Nature of the Internal Work of the Analyst?

What kind of internal work does the analyst do and how does this influence his work with the patient? Can we see evidence of receptivity, patience, and the capacity to allow meaning to cohere without coercion, even within the disruptiveness and turbulence of a first encounter? Is there evidence of reverie, that which we might call a capacity for "dreaming," one avenue for the analyst to encompass the patient's psychic pain and begin to give it meaning? Do we see a difference in the analyst's receptivity to the patient between the first and subsequent meetings? What is the nature of this difference and do we think it indicates something about the analyst's reverie between meetings? Is

there trust enough in this dyad for curiosity and emergent meaning? Is the internal work of the analyst more in the realm of "surviving" than in reflective thought, and what, if anything, does that indicate about the patient, and/or the analytic couple? How do we understand how the analyst accomplishes this "survival?" It will of course be important to check your hypotheses about how the analyst works and his or her internal work by discussing them with the analyst. (Maxine Anderson, William Glover, and Nancy H. Wolf, NAWPIP)

4.4 How Do We See the Patient Responding to How the Analyst Works?

This question naturally refers both to the patient's overt, conscious responses and to what you think you can infer about the patient's unconscious processes. For example, what does this material reveal about the patient's intrapsychic functioning? What does it suggest about the patient's ability to use the analyst and/or the analytic setting? Can you see psychic movement in the patient's responses? How would you describe it? Alternatively, what does not change? Is the movement, if any, related to the psychoanalytic process, and how? What kind of difficulties would you anticipate this patient having in beginning a psychoanalytic process? Once again, we ask you to find evidence for your observations based on the process material and your discussion of it with the analyst.

4.5 How Would You Describe the Nature of This Group's Internal Work?

How have your emotional responses to the material informed your thinking about the initial encounter? How do you perceive the group has received the material and worked with it? Have you observed parallel process phenomena? Has a deepening "meaning space" emerged? Please share the internal experiences and group observations upon which you base your thinking. (Maxine Anderson, William Glover, and Nancy H. Wolf, NAWPIP)

6

WORKING PARTY ON "FAIMBERG'S METHOD FOR THE GROUP DISCUSSION OF CLINICAL MATERIAL

'Listening to Listening'"[1,2]

Haydee Faimberg (Paris), Cláudio Laks Eizirik (Porto Alegre), Sergio Lewkowicz (Porto Alegre)

Introduction

This chapter presents an historical overview of the evolution of "Faimberg's method 'Listening to Listening'", describes its main characteristics and its development in several analytic cultures and concludes with a clinical example of how it works with a group of analysts.

Historical Evolution of the Method as Shaped by the Recognition of Otherness in Intercultural Psychoanalytical Exchanges

On becoming president of the European Psychoanalytical Federation in 2001, David Tuckett had the idea of setting up a Working Party to discuss clinical material and another Working Party to address theoretical issues.

Haydee Faimberg had the privilege of chairing this EPF first Working Party on clinical issues. The task that was established consisted in developing a method that could be used as a way of beginning to talk about clinical material in groups.

DOI: 10.4324/9781032656311-6

Two specific guidelines were followed – and continue to be followed: (a) the group discussion would be predicated on premises that would be different from those underpinning supervisory methods; (b) the way of thinking about the method must be preserved from any temptation to be inspired by an idealized leader, called by Haydee Faimberg an idol (real or imagined).

As Chair, Haydee Faimberg proposed that the various EPF psychoanalytical societies and groups investigate what type of ideas they favoured (both in training and in debates with experienced analysts). The aim was to arouse curiosity as to *the filiation of certain ideas that are taken for granted, that circulate in society, that are taught in the institute and that are passed on as being self-evident without any questions being asked about where the ideas came from or whether any author or authors have proposed them . . .*[3]

The first to initiate an approach along these lines were analysts at the C. Musatti Centre in Milan of the Italian Psychoanalytical Society (SPI) who, during Laura Ambrosiano's term as scientific secretary, put to the vote this proposal for the 2003/2004 scientific programme and adopted a project to study the influences exercised by various authors whom they identified with the analytical approach of the analysts at the Centre. The analysts recognized that those authors had influenced their way of working. The findings of the study were presented in a plenary of the EPF/FEP in Helsinki in 2004. Many clearly interested participants attended, among whom was Cláudio Laks Eizirik, who since that time has alternated as participant and presenter and, in the last few years, as co–coordinator for Latin America with Sergio Lewkowicz, who first participated in 2008 in Vienna.

We always make it very clear that we respect the work of supervision, which we consider to fulfil a different function from that of the dialogue that we were proposing. Many associations organized clinical teaching seminars inspired by that experience of the Working Party, which complemented supervisions. For several years running, colleagues from Australia, Canada, the United States and Latin America attended, in addition of course to those from EPF.

The following year a Panel meeting was organized by German analysts who were profoundly marked by the thinking of Wolfang Loch. It was in that very Panel that we discovered that the cutting of sessions, which we introduced somewhat belatedly in our Working Party (probably in 2003), was practised by Loch and Michel Balint.

This, we think, offers an excellent confirmation that such cutting is *conducive to the co-creation of a discussion time without preconceived certainties*. (We learned later that Meltzer had also applied this technique.) They applied it by cutting before interpretation. This is not how we proceed, but our approach merits a paper in its own right.

The work of cutting entails dividing into segments the presentation of the session. This places the group in the same position of not knowing how the session continues, which is the same position that the presenter had with his patient. This allows time to reflect in the group, and to begin to learn a *language in common . . . to understand differences*.

This type of research into the *filiation of ideas and schools of psychoanalysis* makes it possible to reconstruct and understand the dynamics of how ideas travel, through transmission in personal analysis, in training seminar presentations, in supervisions, in international meetings, through migrations of psychoanalysts.

On the basis of this invaluable experience, Haydee Faimberg started wondering how analysts around the world, in the context of their own culture and at the same time in their singularity, addressed essential psychoanalytical problems, which she, for her part, *could start formulating for herself*.

Recognition of the debt that we owe in the transmission of psychoanalysis forms part of the focus of our investigation, which we continue to pursue today on the basis of the experience thus opened up through the first Working Party which, as we noted, was born in the European Federation (2001–2005).

After that date (2005), in the European Federation Haydee Faimberg preferred to go on working outside the context of a working party, to allow her to recognize from which she was creating what finally became *Faimberg's method listening to listening* (always for the purpose of discussing clinical material in a group).

As she herself put it:

When I speak of basic assumptions I give all credit for this concept to Bion, who was the first to introduce it: that at least was where my concept of basic assumption originated.

A long parenthesis is necessary here: I used the concepts I had created for the clinical situation – in which I always without exception use the psychoanalytical method – and extended those concepts to another field: it is in this new field and

145

only in this new field that I speak of "Faimberg's method 'listening to listening.'"

In other words, as I must stress again because it is essential, the basic concepts through which I contributed personal psychoanalytical ideas, when they are used in the clinical session *are never transformed into a method* that would be substituted for the psychoanalytical method. *When the same concepts are broadened to be used in another field, then it is recognized that it is only here that a method has been created and my name indicates that is structured by personal concepts that originated in the clinical experience.* In a nutshell then, the word *method* here has a different status than the term *psychoanalytical method.* End of parenthesis.

It is to be recalled that the Working Party was intended not to have a supervisory role and not to seek to conform to a real or imaginary ideal model that would prevent us from creating our own *authentic* way of working in analysis.

Some of Haydee Faimberg's inspiration came from previous experiences of intra- and intercultural encounters: partly inspired by the Westpoint and London encounters for the 75th anniversary of the IJPA, she conceived and organized the Conference on Psychoanalytical Intracultural and Intercultural Dialogue (Paris 1998, IPA). She also drew on the model of the annual Franco-British Conference proposed by Anne-Marie Sandler, which Haydee Faimberg had the privilege of cochairing with her (1994–2004) – a conference which continues to this day (still for the discussion of clinical material).

Setting Up the First Working Party's Groups for 2001

In short, our current Working Party grew out of this first Working Party on clinical issues, set up from 2001 to 2005 in the European Federation (EPF/FEP).

The challenge was to set up groups with both open-minded and intellectually demanding colleagues, capable of listening with interest and curiosity to other colleagues. It is difficult to imagine that at that time there was no significant textbook addressing these issues.

Ten groups were set up, each composed of twelve participants. For each group, two moderators were selected (essential), along with one rapporteur and ten experienced analysts to give the presentation.

The creativity of the project hinged on the creativity of the analysts participating.

The point was explicitly made to the participants that, *in listening to the clinical presentation, we did not intend to favour any particular school of analysis*. The dialogue was to be predicated on basic assumptions differing from those governing supervision; an effort was to be made not to take the easy way of following the implicit or explicit leadership of some idol who might be thought to be able to save us from thinking about what was *unknown*.

Our dialogue would be directed specifically towards *discovering – to the extent that we could achieve it – why the presenter worked in the way that he worked*.

Little by little we became able to mutually allow ourselves to "think our ways of thinking" and, instead of a single method that we had initially imagined to be unique, **we came to realize** that we could accept the adventure of imagining that there are *different ways of thinking about the method itself* (just as there are different ways of proceeding in the psychoanalytical session, as we were seeing experimentally in the groups).

As two different styles were already beginning to be there, two strands were organized in this first working party on clinical issues from the second year:

> Strand 1 was directed by David Tuckett in respect of his own style. After 2005 it became the Working Party on clinical comparative methods.
> Strand 2 was the context in which Haydee Faimberg initiated and became able to create from her own perspective the method we are presenting in this chapter, while she continued as Chair of the Working Party on clinical issues at EPF up to 2005.

Haydee Faimberg's modelling in Strand 2 of the method within the framework of the Working Party was informed by one of her main interests, which relates to the way that *one culture understands how another culture addresses essential psychoanalytical problems*.

We reproduce in the following the text setting out "*Faimberg's method listening to listening*" as included in programmes of EPF, IPA, FEPAL[4] and other institutions and sent out as a letter from the Chair to future participants.

Letter from the Chair presenting Faimberg's method listening to listening, for the group discussion of clinical material (to be sent to participants and as it appears in the programmes)

"*While attempting to develop new ways of approaching our discussion on clinical issues, it seems inevitable that at the same time as psychoanalysts we keep in mind our constructs (we cannot not have a theory). It would be an illusion to imagine that we fully understand the basic assumptions of the presenter (underlying his particular way of working) by translating into our own psychoanalytical language what the presenter is trying to convey. **Each analyst/ translator has his own basic assumptions with which he translates.***

We shall go on with the task of co-creating a language to discuss differences and understand the presenter's work.

*More often than we think clinical material is heard from **one** chosen implicit basic assumption (recognized or not).*

*It is part of our goals to train ourselves in listening not only to recognize the presenter's clinical assumptions but also to recognize **our** assumptions as well.*

We shall try to understand from which theory we are listening to the presenter as well as trying to understand from which theory the presenter is listening to his patient and interpreting or not interpreting. We explore the impact that the theoretical assumptions of each participant have on the discussion itself.

In this kind of dialogue we would be using the function of 'listening to listening' which I had initially limited to the psychoanalytical listening in the session [Faimberg, 1981]. That is, to listen to how each intervention in the discussion of the group is heard by the others in a particular context of the discussion.

*From the gap existing between what the participant thought he was saying and how he was heard we begin to co-create a language to understand the psychoanalytical complexity of each issue. By 'listening to how each participant listens to each other', the sources of **misunderstanding** may appear and we thus begin to recognize the basic assumptions of each participant (which might indeed be at the origin of the misunderstanding).*

Accordingly, listening to misunderstanding is a valuable tool for discovering different implicit basic assumptions.

This method, this style of discussion, has its own logic, its own coherence, which we shall seek to develop to the fullest possible extent.

Allow me to stress at the risk of repeating myself that the aim of the common language we wish to create is to understand how each person works in a different way and why a particular analyst works as he/she does. It is not at all the aim to appreciate the other because he is just like 'me', but to know in what way he is different. Different in the sense of recognizing his/her different basic assumptions; not different for what 'I' think the differences are in relation solely to my own basic assumptions. Common language refers therefore to a way of understanding each other in the group, not to a project of working as psychoanalyst in a similar way.

Though it might seem a difficult task, I feel it does justice to differences rather than idealizing sameness.

The fact that the criteria for recognizing differences are developed in the actual practice of the method does not mean that the method does not in itself have clear goals. The goal clearly set by the method is to discover why an analyst (the presenter) works as he does. And this discovery changes from one presentation to another, as discussed in the group by virtue of this method. The clear goal of making **new** discoveries derives from the method itself.

The analyst presents the sessions, divided in sequences, so that in each sequence the group can discuss from the position of not-knowing what happens afterwards (which was the original position of the presenter as analyst).

We take the time to reflect on links between modes of working and underlying basic assumptions. It is important to use all the time allowed for the exchange. The group is composed of about 20 members (included the presenter and moderators)."

We propose to read before participating in one of the groups the following bibliography:

Faimberg, H. "Listening to listening" (1981), "Misunderstanding and psychic truths" (1995), "Narcissistic Discourse as a Resistance to Psychoanalytical Listening: A Classic submitted to the test of Idolatry", Chapters 7, 8 and 9 in Haydee Faimberg *The Telescoping of Generations: Listening to the Narcissistic Links between Generations*, London and New York: Routledge 2005.

Faimberg, H. (2019) "Basic theoretical assumptions underpinning Faimberg's method

'Listening to listening'", *International Journal of Psychoanalysis*, Vol. 100, 3, 447–462.

We shall now talk about the background to our choosing to present our current Working Party by way of this text and the publication of "Basic assumptions underpinning Faimberg's method: Listening to listening" in the *International Journal* (2019).

First Working Party to Discuss
Clinical Issues (EPF/FEP) 2001–2005

(a) What Haydee Faimberg Did Not Know . . . . as Yet

At that time she was not *as yet* (Faimberg, 2013a) clearly aware that she was looking for a method centred on *recognizing what were the basic assumptions of the person who was presenting clinical material and how much they shaped that person's way of working.*

*She did not know that this method would actually consist in **inferring** from the presenter's way of working **what were those basic assumptions** (and especially the implicit ones). She did not know that we would ask the presenter to participate as he wished, taking particular care not to talk prematurely about his **explicit** basic assumptions in order to facilitate the proper unfolding of this kind of dialogue (in which the presenter participates).*

Haydee Faimberg did not know as yet that she was going to pay special attention to the ***misunderstanding*** that would (*inevitably*) arise in our dialogue. This would necessarily be so, since when one person (with certain basic assumptions) listened to another person (with different basic assumptions), it could logically be deduced that *what was said and what was listened to would not be sure to coincide.*

She was still unaware that when in a discussion this misunderstanding was not able to be recognized, an effort needed to be made to be able to listen to what was being listened to on either side, and this became a key task for the two moderators.

Haydee Faimberg was still unaware that clinical concepts she had created would need to be taken up again because she had developed them only for the situation with the patient. Now she had made use of them again at another level, namely, in order to construct a method for listening to analysts who work in a different way and to be able to recognize as exactly as possible where the difference lies.

To appreciate the complexity of each concept we invite the reader interested in the subject to read:

(in relation to the whole concepts underpinning this method) Faimberg 2019 (pages 452–453); (with reference to the concepts of "listening to listening") (Faimberg, [1981] 2005); (in relation to a basic concept used in the dialogue in the group to discover all the participants [including the presenter of course], namely, "misunderstanding" (Faimberg, [1995] 2005); "recognition of otherness" (Faimberg, [1981] 2005) and the "as yet situation" (Faimberg, 2013a).

Haydee Faimberg did not suspect that when, on a great many occasions, such an experience occurred (and constituted so many turning points in the discussion), it would often be **the presenter who would prove to be curious and stimulated by the possible discovery of what was unknown through the dialogue . . . even though the clinical material was what** *he himself was presenting* !

Haydee Faimberg did not suspect that she would even look for an unspoken active misunderstanding if she had not yet encountered it, particularly at certain times when no one wished to say anything that would reveal any difference with the presenter. The intense desire to build on a *fraternal collaboration seemed at times to be paid for by an inhibition to recognize differences.*

Our experience revealed the relief felt by the protagonists when in these circumstances *creative access is obtained to something that was not previously identified, and realizing that this discovery is different from what we usually think, that it is discovered with surprise, may translate into an extraordinary movement of cohesion to look for differences and create a feeling of high esteem within the group.*

"On this basis, wanting to know why the presenter works as he does becomes a genuine subject of **investigation**" (Faimberg, 2019, p. 458). In other words, in our model the investigation is made *in the group by way of the method. This is our method of investigation.*

(b) The as Yet Situation, the Psychoanalytical Method as a Frame[5]

What Haydee Faimberg indeed knew *was that the criterion of working like or not working like each of the participants could not be used as the **only**criterion for listening and discussing.*

She knew that she did not want to apply a known theory and to recognize it in the presenter's way of working. She did not want to listen to only what we expected to listen to.

Only later could she think that "*instead of steering clear of misunderstandings, we listen for a particular kind of understanding which offers us a path to recognizing a polyphony of basic assumptions, This is very different from considering a misunderstanding merely as a sound that rings false, that we must correct, a sound emitted by mistake in a (non-existent or illusory) concord of sound".*

Without these basic assumptions, the method proposed could not continue to be the method that it is and that is designed for the "hunting" of psychoanalytical thought, including its unconscious dimension.

(Faimberg, 2019, p. 460)

The Faimberg's Method
Listening to Listening in Latin America

After its initial introduction and development in Europe, the Faimberg's method listening to listening was extensively applied in Latin America. On several occasions, Haydee Faimberg and Antonio Corel chaired groups using what was initially called the "listening to listening" method. The APA Diccionario contains the following entry, under "método" ("method"): "Método Faimberg escucha de la escucha" ("Faimberg´s method listening to listening") (See footnote 1). This method has been identified by the same name in FEPAL since the Presidency of Luis Fernando Orduz (2014–2016).

During several visits to Latin America, where they took part in all FEPAL congresses from 2006 on, as well as visiting different societies, in Porto Alegre they developed an intense clinical and theoretical programme and chaired groups, jointly with Cláudio Laks Eizirik and Sergio Lewkowicz, using the method. Thereafter, following this immersion of the majority of members and candidates in the method, Eizirik and Lewkowicz began chairing groups that used this original, ground-breaking approach. A growing number of invitations followed, and subsequently these two analysts have worked regularly at all FEPAL and FEBRAPSI congresses, chairing groups using the Faimberg's method listening to listening, as well as working with Faimberg, Corel and Dieter Burgin at all IPA congresses in their pre-congress programmes. The work of Haydee Faimberg was also drawn on in the training of candidates and it is applied in several societies. In recent years, Eizirik and Lewkowicz have been invited to apply the method in different countries and cities, including Rio, São Paulo, Fortaleza, Campo Grande, Sao José do Rio Preto, Marília, Uberlândia, Ribeirão Preto, Porto Alegre, Montevideo, Buenos Aires, Asuncion and Lima.

This Latin American outreach is a work in progress, and it seems to us that this is a frequently sought and widely accepted way of improving psychoanalytic listening and the ability of analysts to learn how to listen to others, to themselves and to patients. *Faimberg's method listening to listening* offers the possibility, precisely through listening to listening, of exploring and identifying the basic assumptions of the participants and of the presenter and fruitfully identifying misunderstandings. Sometimes, we observe that the immersion of the group in the method also gives rise to a kind of reliving or enactment of the analytic field and expressions of transference, countertransference and fantasies of the original session. These moments are useful to explore listening to listening, the misunderstandings and the emotional atmosphere of the session (Eizirik et al., 2016).

An important development inspired also by the Faimberg's method listening to listening was the establishment, in the IPA, in 2005, of CAPSA (Committee on Analytic Practice and Scientific Activities), during the presidency of Cláudio Laks Eizirik, with the objective of improving clinical practice, particularly the development of psychoanalytic theories and techniques derived from the clinical process and the need for inter-regional exchange of ideas on clinical and related issues.

Working Party on Faimberg's Method Listening to Listening: Listening to Listening for Significant Sequences That Never Recur in the Same Way

No matter where in the three regions the discussion occurs and notwithstanding the unique nature of each group of participants and of the clinical material presented, the kinds of dialogues that take place in the different groups reveal a number of common features, which never recur in the same way. We will now describe some of the discussions in one of these groups, without getting into the specifics of the clinical material, for reasons of confidentiality.

As we have suggested, we seek to give special attention to the impact of *each **participant's basic** assumptions* on how he engages in the discussion.

In the first day of work, after the presentation of some fragments, one participant, expressing his views, says he hears a massive projective identification in the way the analysand speaks to his analyst. Another participant, for his part, comments on the material in a way that can be considered to reflect his basic assumption that projective identification had operated as a way of communication. The moderator and other participants might have thought of something along the lines suggested by Bion (that projective identification may also be a way of communication, Bion, 1962), but may not have said so in order to guard against Bion being transformed into an ideal figure ("an idol", in the words of Haydee Faimberg in a presentation of a paper in 2001,[6] in the EPF) who would thus **be used in different ways to** block further dialogue within the *space thus created by the method.*

Within the group in question, a friendly atmosphere reigns, at least on the surface. At this point (as he noted on the second day), a third member of the group is inwardly critical of the absence of any reference to the concept of defence, but "prefers" not to mention it to the group, to ward off any dissension. (We are reminded by this that no criticism was voiced during certain presentations and that unspoken criticism was expressed outside the meeting. This was one of the situations the method takes care to overcome, with the aim of discussing within the group instead of displacing any criticism to the corridors. . . .

This situation reflects the fact that the whole discussion is perhaps implicitly ruled by one basic assumption: *the criterion of "working like me or not working like me". At that moment, that criterion is used not just to compare differences in our minds (as a first step towards finding our familiar points of reference), but as the **only** criterion for listening to and discussing the clinical material presented. In other words, this criterion **alone** is used as the way of deciding whether the work is good (if he works like me); if he works differently, I consider that he is not a good analyst.* It is difficult to accept difference, it is difficult to listen to and recognize *otherness.* This is precisely the task of this kind of discussion. Differences are not a given; discussion in the group gradually creates a common language and then makes it more and more possible to recognize differences, to accept them as such, to recognize, in short, otherness.

On the second day an apparently friendly dialogue seems to suggest some measure of agreement. We then see an example of an interesting kind of dialogue – one, however, that never occurs in the same way and is *never anticipated.*

The third member of the group feels somehow more reassured and so is emboldened to express his views. He asks why the analyst did not even once analyze the defences. In the dialogue it becomes clearer and clearer that behind this insistent question lies an important basic assumption on the part of this participant (and which the rest of the group begins to hear as what we call "a misunderstanding"). This participant's basic assumption is that we should *always* first interpret the defences, thus implicitly suggesting that the presenter was not working in the *right* direction. We could think (**perhaps not all the members at the same time and not all meaning it in the same way**) that there had been a danger all the time in the minds of the participants on the first day that the friendly discussion . . . had failed.

Then something happened that rendered the danger less dangerous, so to speak, because the presenter became able to say that, *reflecting now on that dialogue*, it was clearer to him that he had in mind the notion of resistance, and not the notion of defences. A lively discussion then ensued, which seemed to many of us an *authentic* friendly exchange on the differences between the two approaches: the group (moderator, presenter and the other analysts) *began to try to reconstruct the source* of what clearly was considered a "misunderstanding": the presenter thought that at that moment the patient was **not resisting the analytic work**. To the question as to what the presenter meant by this expression (of not resisting the analytic work), he answered that the patient was associating new and meaningful "material" (so to speak), so there was no resistance. They began to discuss what difference existed between defence and resistance. Accordingly, the participant who invoked the need to interpret defences *realized that he had all that time been translating in relation, so he said, to his basic assumption that the defences of the ego are the first aim of an interpretation.*

It is interesting to note that when the group does not recognize that there has been a misunderstanding and is less able to consider the source of the misunderstanding to lie in different basic assumptions, **another participant begins to mention important analysts. It became clear to the moderator that *more than one participant* felt the need to seek the "magical" help of an author who was *invoked in that moment as an "idol"*** . These moments are extremely frequent, and they illustrate how, in each group, the Faimberg's method listening to listening makes it evident how often *we all look for such help,* instead of going on to think each in our own different ways about *facing the unknown.* The basic assumptions *of the participants* are thus becoming to be identified, but it is also important to consider then how, once they have been recognized, these basic assumptions help us *then* to begin or continue to try to recognize the *presenter's* basic assumptions.

This is what happens in a group like the one we have described when the presenter becomes curious about the importance he discovers in the group discussion that the basic assumption of resistance has been having in all his work, and starts to listen to in a decentred listening.

The aim thus pursued – which appears in almost all the groups – led us to think that the idol function seemed to be designed to "solve" (in an illusory way) this kind of *as yet situation.*

To sum up what we have said, there is often a moment when the presenter becomes curious about his/her own presentation, and decentres his/her own listening, listens with a different way of listening to the others . . . and poses new questions about the session already presented **. . . as though he/she had not been the presenter.** At this stage, there is a turning point, and the process of listening to listening occurs within the participants' minds, including in particular the presenter who becomes curious to explore his/her own presentation. *This is a moment when the "listening to listening" method works to the best advantage of the group.*

Let us underline that one essential aim of the method is to hold a clinical discussion in a group in the frame of an "as yet situation", a basic assumption of Haydee Faimberg (originally designed for the clinical situation) that concerns *psychic temporality.* It refers to the situation that has not *as yet* happened, up to the moment we begin to discover, with surprise, the *presenter's basic assumptions* when working with his patient. In other words, when we recognize why an analyst – who is presenting the sessions – works as he/she works.

This is by the same token the moment when we recognize that we have become able to overcome the general tendency to listen to clinical presentations on the basis of a privileged and unique theoretical perspective (whether or not recognized as such).

The idea of creating this method has been that the *method itself* creates the conditions to facilitate the most interesting moments of *investigation.*

Notes

1 In the APA Dictionary the keyword "*método*" ("method") has an entry on "Método Faimberg 'escucha de la escucha'" ("Faimberg's method 'listening to listening'". In C. Borensztein (Ed.), *Diccionario del Psicoanálisis Argentino*. Buenos Aires: Editorial APA, 2014a].

2 The IPA Working Party on Faimberg's method: Listening to Listening is composed of Haydee Faimberg, Chair; Dieter Bürgin and Antoine Corel (Europe); Cláudio Laks Eizirik, Sergio Lewkowicz and Victoria Korin (Latin America).

3 In a chapter (Faimberg, 2013b) containing an updated version of her paper on the concept of the countertransferential position (for listening and interpreting), Haydee Faimberg realized that in the Argentine Psychoanalytical Association concepts were being circulated on countertransference that originated unquestionably from Heinrich Racker and that had already been integrated into the Argentine style. Racker died at the young age of 51, so that she and those of the rising generation did not know him personally. *Retroactively, Haydee Faimberg reproached herself for not having wondered enough about the origin of this understanding of the concept of countertransference so characteristic of the analytical style in Argentina.* Subsequently, in the aforementioned chapter, she was able to wonder about how to understand the reference to countertransference in an article by Freud and also in Lacan's conception of the desire of the analyst and the concept of countertransference. But that is another story . . .

4 In each IPA congress our Working Party works in English and in Spanish. As we shall see further on, in FEPAL, following its initial establishment and development in Europe, the method is extensively used. It has *also* become a way of teaching psychoanalysis to candidates in some institutes. Haydee Faimberg and Dieter Burgin regularly chair meetings for Candidates of IPSO and OCAL in International Conferences.

5 Faimberg (2013a, 2014b).

6 Faimberg [2001] 2005.

Bibliography

Bion, W. (1962). A theory of thinking. *International Journal of Psycho-Analysis*, *43*, 306–310.

D. W. Winnicott, Fragment of an Analysis in Tactics and Techniques in Psychoanalytic Therapy, Science House ed. (1972) pp. 455–693.

Eizirik, C. L., Lewkowicz, S., Crestana, T., & Barison, O. (2016). Um exercício de pesquisa clínica em psicanálise: o método Faimberg de escuta da escuta. IPA, II Conferência Regional- As Várias Faces da Pesquisa Clínica, São Paulo.

Faimberg, H. "Listening to listening" (1981), "Misunderstanding and psychic truths" (1995). "Narcissistic discourse as a resistance to psychoanalytical listening: A classic submitted to the test of idolatry", Chapters 7, 8 and 9 in Haydée Faimberg. *The Telescoping of Generations: Listening to the Narcissistic Links between Generations.* Routledge (Original work published 2005).

Faimberg, H. (2012a). José Bleger y su encuadre dialéctico: vigencia actual. In *Calibán. Revista Latinoamericana de Psicoanálisis* (Vol. 10, n. 1, pp. 193–203). Fepal. (Original work published 2012).

Faimberg, H. (2012b). José Bleger's dialectical thinking. *The International Journal of Psychoanalysis, 93,* 981–992; in Portuguese Livro Anual de Psicanálise (XXIV), 2014; in Spanish: "El Pensamiento dialéctico de José Bleger." el Libro Anual de Psicoanálisis, 2013.

Faimberg, H. (2013a). The as yet situation in winnicott's fragment of an analysis (1955): "Your father did not do you the honor of . . . yet". *The Psychoanalytic Quarterly, 82* (4), 849–875.

Faimberg, H. (1992). Chapter 4, The Contratransference Position and the Contertransference in The Telescoping of Generations: Listening to the Narcissistic Links between Generations. London/New York Routledge, 2005.

Faimberg, H. (1993) Misunderstanding and psychic truths, pre-published papers, *International Journal of Psychoanalysis.*

Faimberg, H. (2014a). "Método Faimberg 'escucha de la escucha'" ("Faimberg's method: 'listening to listening'"), [entry "método", "method"]. In C. Borensztein (Ed.), *Diccionario del Psicoanálisis Argentino (Argentine Dictionary of Psychoanalysis).* Editorial APA.

Faimberg, H. (2019). Basic theoretical assumptions underpinning Faimberg's method: "Listening to listening". *International Journal of Psychoanalysis, 100* (3), 447–462.

Fenichel, O. (1945). *119 Rundbriefe (1934–1945).* Stroemfeld Verlag. (Original work published 1998).

Eizirik e-mail: cleizirik@gmail.com
Faimberg e-mail: h.faimberg@gmail.com
Lewkowicz e-mail: sergio.lewkowicz@gmail.com

THE WORKING PARTY "MICROSCOPY OF THE ANALYTIC SESSION"

Developing the Capacity for Clinical Investigation (Dreaming, Interpreting, Validating and Theorizing)

Roosevelt M. S. Cassorla,[1] Ana Clara Duarte Gavião,[2] Cláudia Aparecida Carneiro[3]

Scientific dialogue between psychoanalysts tends to be difficult due to the fact that we are dealing with a complex system of knowledge which may be conceived in distinct ways by various thinkers. This difficulty is reinforced by the inevitable trauma that arises from coming into contact with the Other. On the other hand, it may also be noted that this communication becomes easier in the presence of clinical material. Through dealing with observable facts – albeit in different ways – the clinic enables professionals to pursue paths that stimulate productive agreements and disagreements.

As teachers at institutes of psychoanalysis, our aim is to stimulate the development of the candidates' analytic capacity, expanding the potential for investigation in the clinic. This development would be influenced by creative clinical dialogue with colleagues and, evidently, with themselves. Through trial and error, we have been developing a group-based clinical working technique that is best suited to our candidates and teaching objectives. The result has been the Working Party (WP) named "Microscopy of the Analytic Session."[4]

DOI: 10.4324/9781032656311-7

We start from the premise that developing the capacity to learn through clinical experience can be evaluated through the observation of the vicissitudes of "dreaming," in the sense used by Bion (1962, 1992). Dreaming goes on 24 hours a day just as other biological functions do, such as breathing and digestion. Dreaming is a "theater that generates meanings" (Meltzer, 1983, p. 46). The content of permanent unconscious dreaming is manifest through daydreams and nocturnal dreams. These dreams, in turn, are constantly re-dreamed, and the symbolic network and the capacity to think more abstract thoughts is expanded (Cassorla, 2012).[5]

As outlined later in this chapter, the WP constitutes a process of "dreaming field." The process is triggered by clinical material from sessions that have already taken place. This material creates emotional reverberations in the field, resulting in group dreams that require new ways of thinking. The investigator takes part in the process while also observing it. We are confronted with the psychoanalytic method whose double-sided nature indicates the concomitance of investigation and practice. The investigation also reveals how the teaching-learning process develops. This investigation can also be carried out in other ways, as we will demonstrate later. The description of the functioning of the WP may be accompanied from Item 3 onwards and details the aspects mentioned earlier.

Objectives

1. The principal **Objective** of the WP is to develop the capacity to practice and think about the psychoanalytic clinic.
2. The Specific Objectives follow:
   a. To develop the intuitive capacity of the participants
   b. To develop the capacity for thinking about the phenomena experienced
   c. To develop the capacity for constructing interventions/ interpretations, including the paths that lead to this
   d. To identify and understand implicit and explicit theories that guide the analytic work
   e. To develop the capacity for validation of the clinical work
   f. To develop the capacity for clinical investigation

The WP permits the investigation of other Specific Objectives depending on the ways in which the material is studied.

Theoretical Assumptions

The coordinators use the following theoretical assumptions or hypothetical models to guide their observation:

1. The WP member's ensemble constitutes a group in which there is the installation of a field (Baranger & Baranger, 1961–1962), the WP field, in which group members influence each other. Nothing occurs with any member that does not reverberate in the others. The clinical material and the analyst who presents the material also influence the members.

2. The concept of field leads observers to pay less attention to facts than to the relationships and influences that exist among them. The phenomena occurring in the WP field are transitory and constantly changing. The observer influences them, and they modify the observer as well. Their apprehension, which occurs whenever they move, is punctual, and, while they are apprehended, they have already changed.

3. The WP field is considered a "dream's" field (Cassorla, 2016). This model considers that the emotional experiences occurring in the WP seek transformation into images – like waking dreams – which, in turn, are connected to words. The field will reveal both the dreams symbolized by words and also facts seeking symbolization (non-dream) that are revealed by emotions, discharges, acts, and other forms of non-thought.

4. Each intervention made by a group member is seen as an emergent of the field that reveals its dynamics in that exact moment. The WP field functioning is considered analogous to the mind functioning. The adopted model of the mind implies unpredictable connection possibilities between aspects with varying degrees of symbolization and non-symbolization. It also involves attacks on both the possibilities of connection and the connections already established. The symbolic and non-symbolic facts include affective aspects that involve and are surrounded by them. In this model, the mind is the outcome of other minds' fertilization, which in turn are fertilized by it.

161

5. In the analytic field, the analyst's interventions result from the negotiation between intuited aspects and thought about these aspects; the analyst working with the patient does this task consciously and unconsciously. The interventions are the culmination of this negotiation that includes the dreams being dreamed and non-dreams that are looking for dreamers. The same occurs in the WP field: a conscious and unconscious negotiation between the intuitions that arise in the field (this field constituted by the interaction among the WP members and other field products).

Technical Procedures

The technical procedures are based on the detailed study of clinical material presented by a colleague.

1. The colleague in charge presents part of a session. The part is interrupted before the analyst intervenes.
2. The group, invited to "dream" the clinical material, discusses freely.
3. Based on the discussion, the "selected facts" (Bion, 1962) of the group are identified, which form the basis for the hypothetical interventions that are proposed to deal with the material presented.
4. The group seeks to identify the implicit theories that have determined the proposed hypothetical interventions.
5. The group listens to the intervention done by the analyst and the sequence of the clinical material. Possible implicit theories that have determined the analyst's intervention are discussed.
6. The group compares the analyst's intervention, the interventions proposed by the group, and the dynamics of the psychic change (or its absence) in both observation fields (the session and the WP). At this point, facts related to the scientific validation are discussed.
7. Another part of the session is presented, and so on . . .
8. During the activity, at the discretion of the coordinators, the group is encouraged to observe and discuss the group dynamic when faced with the material presented.
9. At the end, the presenting analyst takes the floor and discusses the material and his impressions of the group work.

10. Next, the group evaluates, in detail, the work that has been done. Three or four weeks later, each member responds in writing to questions set by the coordinators.

Each group is composed of approximately 15 psychoanalysts or candidates. Work was conducted for eight to 12 hours. There was a coordinator and one or two co-coordinators, whose functions were defined. The meetings were recorded, and, at the same time, the co-coordinators took notes as they listened. The recording was transcribed and complemented by these notes.

Researchers know that both the addition of participants and the hypotheses formulated by investigators are influenced by conscious and unconscious assumptions. As occurs with the psychoanalyst in his practice, the task of both the analyst and the investigator is to transform their subjective apprehension into something objective. The reader, having access to the material, will be able to formulate their own assumptions.

The type of research proposed requires lengthy texts that make presentation of this material difficult. This text will present, as an illustration, short excerpts from a WP conducted with members and candidates. Although emotions experienced by the group play an extremely important role in the development of the WP's work, unfortunately it is not possible to convey the gamut of these emotions in the excerpts that follow.

First Stage: "Dreaming"

ANALYST: "It's the first session of the week, Monday, 7:30 in the morning, I open the door of the consulting room and find him standing outside, wailing, hugging his briefcase. He comes in and stays standing, crying, he seems not to know what to do. I ask him if he wants to lie down on the couch; he lies down on his stomach and remains in this position for some time, until he turns to me and says: 'Good morning. I'm sorry to present myself in this way. I can't be like this with anyone, not even with you. I almost called to say I wouldn't be able to come, but I came, because I need help. Either I come here, or I throw myself out of the fifth-story window! Because I'm feeling really bad (he cries a lot). I feel like I can't do anything, I don't know how to live a happy life being who I am, there's just no way to fix it!'"

163

COORDINATOR: "You're all free to express your own experiences, communicate your fantasies, dreams, waking dreams."

(The group works for approximately 35 minutes. The following interventions have been edited to summarize.)

The first intervention describes the sensation of helplessness, despair, desolation, "those emotional things." The group associates images and ideas with these "things." A figure is visualized standing on the edge of a precipice looking for a ledge to stop themselves from falling. The ledge is associated with a hug, represented by the briefcase he is holding. The ensuing associations focus on the group's identification with the analyst, who is seen as the protective ledge. The group expresses despair, and the patient's phrases are repeated: "I can't do anything, there's no way to fix it." A feeling of estrangement surfaces, which is then associated with aversion. The group tries to give meaning to this estrangement. Notions of retreating, taking a step backwards, are associated with aversion and despondency. The perception of these aspects continues with feelings of confusion. The group becomes immersed in the details of the issue of confusion/estrangement. Gradually it is observed that the desire to help is accompanied by the sensation there may be threats and manipulation. This is associated with the experience of feeling blackmailed. The "throwing himself out of the fifth-story window" includes despair as well as deceit. The group's impression is that something deceptive is emerging. There is a huge pressure to "grab the hand of someone who is drowning." If this act of saving does not occur, then the guilt will be terrible. The group cites a mixture of feelings: hope, distrust, manipulation, and blackmail. The group goes on to invoke song lyrics, works of literature, and popular sayings that help with the naming of things. Jokes surface that allow the group to breathe. An image appears of a doll that can't stand up, has no energy in its legs, one that is collapsing. The memory of the expression "Good morning!", felt to be false, leads the group to identify other factors for the aversion experienced. The group persists with the perception that it is struggling with contradictory feelings: wanting to "embrace the patient," aversion, and the risk of giving up. An image surfaces of the business executive, wearing his suit and tie like armor and carrying a briefcase with a false bottom that falls apart on opening. It's as if he had no backbone and the couch would have to substitute. The associations lead the group to recall an anecdote about a wedding night where the new groom asks for a room with a strong latch on the window to stop the bride from "throwing herself from the fifth-story."

This stage is interrupted by the coordinator, an intervention which is reluctantly accepted by the group.

COMMENTS FROM THE INVESTIGATORS: At the very beginning of the exercise, there is noticeable progress made in the direction of achieving the proposed objectives. The development of the capacity to "dream" phenomena from the field is evident. The group's functioning is shown to be similar to the functioning of a mind that links together dreams and thoughts by broadening the symbolic network of thinking. The group shows itself to be capable of altering its vertices of observation by seeking to integrate the various experiences it has undergone. Variations in the emotional environment indicate the vitality of the work. The follow-up reporting on the session will demonstrate the congruence, or not, of the underlying hypotheses that manifest within the group.

(They return to reading the material.)

ANALYST: "What do you think needs to be fixed, and what seems to be irreparable?"

(Silence.)

PATIENT: "I'd like to be content with myself, I'm not content, in the relationships I have, mainly with my family, and this weekend I spoke to my Mom, Dad, sister . . . why are some people happy and they don't know it? Because I think so much about existence, and the more I think, the more I ask myself: 'what's happening?'" (He interrupts this thought with another.) "I don't like the couch! Can I sit in the chair?" (He waits for the reaction of the analyst, who suggests that he put himself wherever he prefers.)

At this point, the coordinating team intuits that the work can move on to the second stage: imagining hypothetical interpretations. The beginning of this second part will be transcribed in full.

Second Stage: Hypothetical Interpretations

COORDINATOR: "The next step: you are going to try to imagine what you would say to this patient now. What intervention would you make? Some of you are perhaps thinking, 'I wouldn't say anything; I'd wait a bit longer.' But as part of our exercise, you must tell us what is going through your mind, even if you don't speak to the patient."

(Silence.)

A: (After hesitating over what words to use, concludes:) "Thinking is no substitute for the experience of contact with the other."

B: "I'd talk about changing chairs, and I'd talk about what he's looking for, that he can't seem to find a place where he feels comfortable. I don't know. . . ." (hesitation)

COORDINATOR: "Try to put it into words."

C: ". . . it's difficult to find a place where you feel comfortable."

D: "I think I would say something along the lines of: 'What is happiness, what place is this? Who invented this concept of happiness?' I would not say this critically. But I would say to the patient: 'Where do people find this kind of happiness?'" (laughter).

E: "I thought about how important the modulation of the voice would be for this patient . . . there's terrible pain. I think words are secondary. But the content would be that I'm seeing how he's suffering. . . . 'I'm seeing how you are suffering, but I can also see that you've come here to share this suffering, this pain, with me.'"

F: "I have an intervention. I don't know. . . . 'So you nearly called me to say you weren't going to come, but you came, and you spoke to your mother, your father, and your sister, but I don't know if you feel you were helped by them, you wondered what's happening to you and you come here, you almost didn't come, but you came, and I think that you imagine that, by talking with me, we might be able to understand what's happening to you.' And when he asks: 'can I sit in the chair?' I think he's looking for a place too, in such a way that the analyst might be able to help and clarify what is happening."

(The group thinks this intervention is very long, addressing different aspects at the same time. With the help of the group, the intervention is reworked.)

166

G: "Now I can put it better: 'I think you want me to help you to understand what's happening to you.'"

H: "I would say: 'I see that you're suffering, but you are in great suffering and have come to see me so that I can help you feel better.'"

COORDINATOR: "Based on this material and the group work, six hypothetical suggestions have emerged. There are more that could emerge, but we're going to stop here."

I: "I'd like to make a new suggestion which has only just occurred to me: 'Are you trying to be happy here?'"

Third Stage: Implicit Theories

COORDINATOR: "Now we're going to work on the third step; we're going to leave the clinical part momentarily, and we're going to try to discover which theories have influenced these interpretations, primarily the implicit theories. You are not prohibited from talking about explicit theories . . . according to Lacan, according to Klein or Bion . . . but what will interest us more are the ideas that the analyst used, consciously and unconsciously, which led them to make this intervention.

THE FIRST INTERPRETATION WAS: 'Thinking is no substitute for the experience of contact with the other.'"

J: "I thought the analyst could be thinking about the emotional contact present in the session, between him and the analyst."

K: "I see three points of focus in the interpretation. 'Thinking is no substitute for the experience of some kind of contact . . .' One focus is thinking, thought; another focus is the experience, and maybe the third focus is the other, so it's just one speech which encompasses three points."

COORDINATOR: "And what are the theories behind this? What factors have led them to favor these three aspects, and in this way? You don't have to respond, it's for all of us to think together."

L: "The experience of contact with the other."

M: "I understood that the analyst is trying to think about her own experience, that things are dispersed. How can this be dealt with through thinking? And what is the experience of being with someone in this way? I think she wasn't just saying this to the analysand, she was saying this to herself."

N: "I think there is an invitation for an emotional experience, but I'm asking myself whether it's clear to the patient that it's an invitation. Thinking about the analyst, she speaks 'of the emotional experience.' I'm wondering whether the patient felt more the question of no, of defensiveness, or whether he picked up on the invitation; the invitation is subtler."

COORDINATOR: "How are we going to know what the patient has picked up?"

O: "In the next step."

COORDINATOR: "Exactly, this would be the fourth step, a stage we will be encountering shortly, which is validation. We are going to see what the patient did with the intervention, only the patient is not here. From this point on we will do it with the analyst's intervention. Right now we are going to continue with our own.

But let's observe that there is no interpretation that disagrees with the others, all of them are more or less additional. Which leads us to think that they're all following a close path, which may be right or may be totally wrong, but if it's totally wrong, then the patient will show us, and then we'll see whether the analyst is also following our suggestions" (laughter).

COORDINATOR: "Now we are going to identify implicit theories in the second hypothetical intervention: 'It's difficult to find a place where you feel comfortable!'"

P: "It's a sign that we are not talking about a physical place, a chair, a couch, but rather something about his own skin. . . . It could even be about identity, a true identity . . . it could be sexual . . . one person separated from another . . . feeling comfortable in one's own skin."

The transcript is interrupted. The group will continue thinking about the implicit theories in this hypothetical intervention and in others.

Fourth Stage: Micro-Validation

We have defined micro-validation as an evaluation of what happens during a session's movements (or during the Working Party's movements). In this model, such an evaluation comes about by observing the emergence (or lack thereof) of ideas, affect, memories, and associations in the field. Such factors tell us that the network of symbolic thought is being extended, that dreams-for-two are alive and operant (Cassorla, 2012). Micro-validation is being carried out from the beginning of the exercise. At each stage we note the expansion of the thinking capacity and the variety of vertices that are contemplated. The emotional atmosphere is one of satisfaction and creativity. As we have seen, the fact that the patient is absent precludes a more accurate evaluation of the hypothetical interpretations that were conducted while observing the associations.

The next stage consists of comparing the hypothetical interventions with the interpretation of the analyst. The group discusses these elements. We will not transcribe this discussion.

This phase ends with the analyst's speech. As we will see, she formulates hypotheses on her own theories which had influenced her interpretation. During her speech she compares her intervention to those advanced by the group.

COORDINATOR: (Asks the analyst to read her intervention again and comment on it.)

ANALYST: "You ask for my help, but you seem to need my permission, needing me to approve or disapprove. You seem to be afraid that I will condemn you, as you have, to being a person you consider detestable."

(She continues.) "I think that my implicit theory is associated with the action of a tyrannical superego. . . . I thought it was interesting that you brought up aspects that converged in protecting his suffering. I was thinking about this when you were making your interventions: 'I can see you are suffering;' 'you said you almost didn't come, but you came'; 'you are suffering terribly, and you came here to alleviate that suffering. . . .' I was surprised, listening to you, to hear that you had a similar feeling. Like you, I was searching for elements to address this huge suffering, which appeared from the moment I opened the door. It was necessary to go down to the bottom of the well, which seemed inaccessible."

(As we have seen, the analyst reveals the congruence between her thinking and the group's proposals, which represents a form of validation.)

(The group continues associating and thinking . . . and the WP continues.)

At the end, the group reflects on the work conducted over the course of the WP. We will not edit this part, but we anticipate that it will be confirmed by the data presented in the fifth stage.

Fifth Stage: Towards a Macro-Validation

As we have noted, approximately one month after the WP, the participants were encouraged to write about their experiences. We also suggested that they recount perceptions of their analytic work that may have been influenced by the WP.

The responses were very similar. They were collated and edited using qualitative research approaches (Turato, 2011). We observe a kind of macro-validation, i.e., "the observation of what goes on during 'second moments' outside a patient's sessions (or the WP activity)" (Cassorla, 2012). As it is beyond the scope of this text to reproduce the broad assessments received, we present next a sample of those comments, which indicates the effects of the WP exercise on the participants.

Results

The participants observe the development of their analytic capacity; they are able to digress and wait: "*I noticed the expansion of my capacity to observe and think, a greater 'psychic availability,' a 'floating thinking' with the possibility of digression.*" They may refine their understanding and perception of the vicissitudes of acquiring their analytical identity: "*I experienced important non-measurable transformations which are processed slowly, an improvement in the capacity to observe from different perspectives, which is fundamental to the construction and maintenance of the analytic identity.*"

The process is influenced by the group work and contact with other cultures: "*The experience shared with colleagues enriches the possibility for thinking about the 'unknown,' and the exchange with professionals from different regions and cultures with different levels of experience produces another kind of knowledge.*"

The proposed exercise combats rigidity of thought and develops listening: "*My work has changed in the way I listen to patients; I have been trying to be more 'without memory,' more liberated from prior conceptions.*" It transforms and symbolizes: "*I can get closer to my patients, reduce my attention to the manifest contents; I am able to dream, to give figurative form, to symbolize.*"

170

The participants are confronted with the complexity and biases of the process: "*It made me think about multiple approaches for the same patient and how analysis functions with different psychoanalysts. . . . A better knowledge of 'where' one is listening from draws our attention to the inevitable biases that interfere with our listening to the patient.*"

The evaluations accentuate the changes perceived in the analytic work and differentiation: "*It enabled some transformations in my way of working . . . the most evident was the broadening of my thinking capacity. . . . They are the best experiences of the congresses. . . . One lives a greater emotional intensity; it is not a theoretical activity and goes beyond a clinical exercise.*"

Discussion and Conclusions

The impossibility of conveying the complexity of the features that make up the investigation is a frustration that is well known to clinical researchers. Explanations, which are added to other methods, are substituted for descriptions and hypotheses which, in turn, are linked to other observations and hypotheses, and so on and so forth. In this study, we observe how this movement takes place in the field of the WP.

Our work has shown the helpfulness of our initial assertion. That is, that emotional experiences stimulated by the presentation of clinical material drive the process of unconscious dreaming, the content of which is manifest in the WP field through daydreams. These dreams, in turn, are constantly re-dreamed, and the symbolic network and the capacity to think is expanded. The connection between the dreams of all members of the group constitutes what we would call dreams-for-n members, as an analogy for the dreams-for-two which take place between patient and analyst. These elements demonstrate how each analyst develops the capacity to investigate his or her clinic.

The value of the group work was evident, and the participants considerably appreciated the opportunity to interact with colleagues from a range of backgrounds and theorizations. The development of the capacity to listen to others stood out within an atmosphere of respect and collaboration.

Undoubtedly, there were moments when the group's dreaming capacity became more difficult, resonating from what originated in the clinical material. In the material studied we highlight moments of despondency, disinterest, estrangement, confusion, euphoria, etc. and any doubts or hesitations involved in putting ideas and feelings into words. However, the group quickly returns to the dream work integrating disparate aspects.

Occasionally, in situations where the group work was paralyzed, the coordinators encouraged the group to identify factors that could be contributing to this.

We are aware that "false dreams" can exist (Cassorla, 2016), in other words, situations in which an apparent broadening of the thinking capacity conceals areas that cannot yet be dreamed. These are usually identified during the work or afterwards.

We consider the stages in which the group is asked to think about hypothetical interventions to be important, that – in succession – hypotheses are formulated on the implicit theories that would influence the choice of these interventions and the subsequent discussion of the processes of validation. In the transcribed text, the group chose to interpret factors related to finding a link to give containment to the experience of suffering, setting aside other hypotheses related to deceit and manipulation. These would return at points during the WP.

We also note that the group became intensely involved during the discussion of the processes of validation. We have the impression that these aspects, although intuited, are not sufficiently considered in the training and practice of psychoanalysts.

It is beyond the remit of this text to discuss the vicissitudes of investigation in psychoanalysis. We agree with the idea that "it is useless to try to find, among scientific models, a method of research in psychoanalysis; its specificity is inseparable from its praxis" (Botella & Botella, 2001, p. 425). Referring back to Freud (1938/1964), these authors remind us that investigation requires the creation of conditions to "test" the experience through its repetition among a large number of analysts. This fact does not prevent us from being able to carry out research studies on psychoanalysis, quantifying observations and the results that emerge from analytic processes.

To address the teaching-learning process that occurs during the analyst's work, our technique prioritized the use of the clinical psychoanalytic method, albeit adapted to new conditions. However, it has also proved useful to study the links made by the participants when the clinical psychoanalytic method was set aside.

172

Observation biases, stemming from personal factors, form part of the investigation. They can be reduced through continued observation of the field, through the exchanges between the various investigators during the exercise and through perspectives gained after it has ended.

The analysis of the participants' reports also has limitations. Twenty percent of the participants did not respond. We assumed that the time that elapsed between the activity and writing the reports would enable less restricted reporting. Although the participants manifested their enthusiasm with the results, we have no way of knowing about the depth and stability of the potential changes.

The value of the method is also confirmed by the fact that its objectives are met in every WP that is conducted, in different ways of course. Its offering as a teaching activity is being discussed by the candidates. WPs are being requested by various societies and groups of psychoanalysts. Many colleagues go on to repeat the experience.[6]

In recent years, we have been investigating what happens when, after detailed discussion of the material, we return to it again from the beginning. Other forms of "second" looks, as we have seen, involve the same material being studied by the same group at a later date, as well as by different groups. Following the participants over long periods would offer interesting insights into their memories of the activity. Another possibility would be to conduct a detailed study of the transcripts made by the members of the original group.

Although it was not our primary objective, we know that the method provides enough material for other investigations of the process. In another text we discuss factors that influence the construction of interpretation (Cassorla et al., 2016). Other ideas include the study of unconscious communication, transformations in the analyst's way of working, comparisons in the psychoanalytic work among analysts from different theoretical fields, etc.

Notes

1 Brazilian Psychoanalytic Societies of São Paulo and Campinas; WP coordinator.

2 Brazilian Psychoanalytic Society of São Paulo; WP co-coordinator.

3 Society of Psychoanalysis of Brasilia; WP co-coordinator.

4 This WP is part of the curriculum at the Institute of the Brazilian Psychoanalytic Society of São Paulo and is recognized by the Brazilian Psychoanalysis Federation (FEBRAPSI) and the Latin-American Psychoanalysis Federation (FEPAL), as it is offered in their congresses.

5 The system of references described involves concepts pertaining to Bion's theory of thinking including the alpha function, container-contained relationship, emotional linking, transformations, etc.

6 We recommend that participants broaden their knowledge by attending other WPs that use different approaches to studying the clinical material.

Bibliography

Baranger, M., & Baranger, W. (2008). The analytic situation as a dynamic field. *International Journal of Psychoanalysis*, *89*, 795–826. (Original work published 1961–62).

Bion, W. R. (1962). *Learning from experience*. Heinemann.

Bion, W. R. (1992). *Cogitations*. Karnac.

Botella, C., & Botella, S. (2001). A pesquisa em psicanálise [Research in psychoanalysis]. In A. Green (Ed.), *Psicanálise contemporânea: Revista Francesa de Psicanálise: Número especial* (pp. 421–442). Imago.

Cassorla, R. M. S. (2012). What happens before and after acute enactment: An exercise of clinical validation and broadening of hypothesis. *International Journal of Psychoanalysis*, *93*, 53–89.

Cassorla, R. M. S. (2016). Dreams and non-dreams: A study on the field of dreaming. In S. M. Katz, R. M. S. Cassorla, & G. Civitarese (Eds.), *Advances in contemporary psychoanalytic field theory: Concept and future development* (pp. 91–110). Karnac.

Cassorla, R. M. S., Gavião, A. C. D., Carneiro, C., Galvani, M. R. P., Silva, M. P., & Carvalho, R. M. L. L. (2016). The construction of interpretation: Investigation performed during the Working Party "Microscopy of the analytic session" [Paper presentation]. IPA Clinical Research Meeting, São Paulo.

Freud, S. (1964). An outline of psycho-analysis. In J. Strachey (Ed. & Trans.), *The standard edition of the complete psychological works of Sigmund Freud* (Vol. 23, pp. 139–208). Hogarth Press. (Original work published 1938).

Meltzer, D. (1983). *Dream-life: Re-examination of the psycho-analytical theory and techniques*. Clunie.

Turato, E. R. (2011). *Tratado de metodologia da pesquisa clínico-qualitativa [Treaty of clinical-qualitative research methodology]*. 5th edition. Vozes.

8

FREE CLINICAL GROUPS – A PEER GROUP-CENTRED METHOD FOR EVALUATING

Options of Interpretation

Claudia Thußbas, Dorothee von Tippelskirch-Eissing, Peter Wegner[1]

Background

Discussing one's clinical work with a group of colleagues has served a valuable function in the psychoanalytic tradition for many years now, especially when older training analysts with a wealth of clinical experience offer their knowhow. Although these opportunities are highly sought after and appreciated, and rightly so, there has also been criticism of the approach. Younger colleagues in particular, who perhaps have to acknowledge that their efforts were misdirected and that other understandings or interpretations would have been more fitting, often end up frustrated, asking "So how on earth did they come up with that interpretation?" This approach thus sometimes results in a kind of pseudo-superiority that does not reflect greater experience, but more the superiority associated with an ascribed role. The presenter goes away frustrated and unlikely to want to present their own work again in the future.

Wolfgang Loch, holder of the first chair dedicated specifically to psychoanalysis in Europe (1971–1982), must have been aware of these mechanisms. While his written work was highly theoretical and firmly embedded in the German philosophical academic tradition, he preferred to use simple, direct, lively, and humorous

DOI: 10.4324/9781032656311-8

language in his clinical work. One of his few works published in English, *The Art of Interpretation: Deconstruction and New Beginning in the Psychoanalytic Process* (published posthumously in 2006), gives an insight into his writing style. Regrettably, the only documentation of his clinical language derives from the passive memories of training analysands, supervisees, and the many participants in his Balint groups and intervision peer groups. Participants in his clinical groups gained direct insights into the handling of unconscious messages and their transformation into contexts of understanding – knowledge that is difficult to acquire theoretically. It was the experience of working with Loch in this context that encouraged Joachim F. Danckwardt, Ekkehard Gattig, and Peter Wegner to build on the idea of there being various "options of interpretation" to develop the Free Clinical Groups (FCG) method. In the first part of this chapter, we give an account of the key steps in this process. In the second part, we describe the method of FCG that is currently offered at the annual conference of the European Psychoanalytical Federation (EPF). In the third part, we use an example from clinical practice to illustrate the approach. Finally, we consider the current significance and future development of the method.

History and Development of Free
Clinical Groups (FCG)

The development of the FCG method was informed by Loch's reports on his experience of the Balint method in London and other publications, as well as by the clinical seminars of Fritz Morgenthaler and by Wegner's research on the meaning of the opening scene in the initial psychoanalytic interview. In the following sections, we retrace these developmental steps of the FCG method.

The Prisma Effect, Options of Interpretation, and the Episode

In winter 1958/59, Wolfgang Loch first participated in seminars with general practitioners that Michael Balint was running in London.

> The aim of the case discussions in these seminars was to diagnose the affective-emotional dynamics of the doctor–patient/patient–doctor relationship, in order to open up a space for therapeutic

influence. This approach was based on the lived experience of many researchers, not only from the psychoanalytic perspective, that affective-emotional relationships have psychically pathogenic outcomes and/or somatogenic effects.

(Loch, 1995, p. 7, own translation)

The main objective of the method was to enable general practitioners to take various diagnostic levels, beyond the purely physical, into account in their dealings with patients, and furthermore, to be able to place psychotherapeutic interventions (see, e.g., Balint, 1964; Loch, 1966; Sklar, 2017). Loch was "deeply impressed" by the method and returned to London at least twice in the following years to attend seminars with Michael Balint, Enid Balint, or Pierre Turquet (Loch, 1995, p. 7). He was particularly interested in the potential of enabling general practitioners to gain access to their patients' inner life. "For wherever the general practitioner succeeds in strengthening the patient's ego through a deft therapeutic intervention, he opens a door to recovery, as the strengthened ego may be able to discard its past neurotic organizations" (Loch, 1966, 1995, p. 31, footnote 7, own translation). The very first Balint seminar in Germany was then initiated in the 1960/61 winter semester in Frankfurt, with Alexander Mitscherlich as leader and Wolfgang Loch as co-leader.

After moving to Tübingen to work with Walter Schulte (head of what was then the University Psychiatric Clinic) in 1964 and being appointed to his own chair of psychoanalysis at the University Clinic in 1971, Loch continued to lead regular Balint groups until after his retirement in 1982. In the 1970s, he invited guests from abroad, especially from London, to Tübingen for lectures on group research (Loch, 1992, p. 227).

At the very beginning of a key article on the practice and problematic issues of Balint groups, Loch (1995) listed the many factors that should be taken into account when considering the functioning of clinical groups: the presenting analyst, the patient, the presentation of case material, the group, and the moderator and co-moderator or group observer – not to mention the interrelations between all of these factors. The material worked on in the groups is not limited to what is said, surmised, or put into words, but also includes everything that is enacted, gesticulated, or performed. It is perhaps due to this inherent complexity that relatively few publications on the functioning of clinical groups are available to date.

Loch (1964, 1972) himself described the *key elements of his version of the method* as follows:

> What then unfolds in the following discussion [i.e., after the "opening scene" has been reported; see Wegner, 1992, p. 290] could be called the *prism effect* of the group. Just as the prism fans the light out into colours, the commentaries of the members of the group reveal the motive-structure of the doctor–patient relationship in its separate elements.[2] In this way, the presenting doctor finds out a great deal about his patient's relationships and responses that he previously overlooked. At the same time, the general discussion gives him direct insights into his own blind spots. Moreover, his colleagues' comments or targeted questions direct him to gaps in his awareness or other countertransferences that may impair his clear judgment. It can also be observed, and in the case of severely disturbed patients it is in fact initially the rule, that all *participants in the seminar* slip into a joint countertransference role, by either identifying with the suffering patient or by producing a reaction formation to the patient's hidden agenda. This leads by way of a psychical *resonance effect* to a mirroring of the patient's psychodynamic condition within the group.
>
> (p. 281, own translation unless noted otherwise)

In contrast to Balint, Wolfgang Loch understood supervision as a group task and developed a group theory for it.

After the 1990 DPV spring conference in Tübingen,[3] Loch's take on the Balint Group method led to the setting up of the "Achalm Seminars" (Haas, 1995, pp. 161f.), which then took place annually:

> The group supervision focuses on the analysis of an 'episode' with the subgoals of (a) becoming attuned to and empathizing with the patient's situation, (b) gaining insights from the reported transference–countertransference constellation into the pathogenic object relationship, (c) comparing the pathogenic object relationship, as reflected in the treatment situation, with the internal and external conflicts experienced in the life history

and (d) finally discussing other possible understandings, alternative options of interpretation, and other ways of therapeutic practice.

(Haas, 1995, p. 161, own translation)

The focus on the "episode" and the acceptance of there being various different options of interpretation were the decisive steps that opened up a new perspective and informed the further development of the method.

The *prism effect* offers a convincing explanation of why diverse comments (of differing tendency, colour, structure, and detail) can complement, extend, or improve the understanding of the situation as a whole. Moreover, a fundamental structural equivalence must be assumed between psychoanalytical processes of exchange in the classic psychoanalytic setting and the setting of a psychoanalytic Balint group or FCG. Were this structural correspondence not given, it would be impossible to explain how such detailed inferences can be drawn in one setting about the other, thus affording new insights into diagnosis and treatment.

The further development of the method consisted in the strict reduction of the material to be presented in the group situation. Two findings by Morgenthaler and Wegner inspired this. These are presented next.

"Emotionality"

In the early 1980s, the Zurich-based psychoanalyst Fritz Morgenthaler began to offer special dream seminars (Morgenthaler, 1986, pp. 149ff.) that became legendary in the German-speaking countries. Besides Morgenthaler's personality, one of the features characterizing the method was that only the dream itself was reported to the group, without the respective associations, biographical information, or details of the treatment process.

If we refrain from factoring in the dreamer's associations and the whole dream situation, then the means that the psychoanalytical method offers for interpreting the dream are better structured, highlighted, like a relief. That is the real purpose of conducting a dream seminar.

(Morgenthaler, 1986, p. 150, own translation)

Two further characteristic features of Morgenthaler's method of conducting dream seminars were that it considered the formal aspects of a dream (as opposed to the content) and concentrated on the emotionality of a patient's/group's experiences (as opposed to any intellectual processes). This bold approach, paring down the material considered to the manifest dream, encouraged us to take a similar approach and to work with much reduced clinical material.

The Opening Scene

From 1986 to 1988, Peter Wegner empirically examined the meaning of the opening scene in the initial psychoanalytic interview, drawing on the work of Loch (episode, prism effect) and Morgenthaler (manifest dream), among others. Wegner (2014a) defined the opening scene as follows:

> The entirety of the interaction that occurs between analyst and patient, from the personal greeting up to the outset of the interview, including the first spoken sentence, under the basic conditions of psychoanalytic treatment that is offered. The 'entirety of the interaction' denotes all the verbal and nonverbal actions, all the direct and indirect communications, as well as all the same accompanying conscious, preconscious and unconscious psychic processes [cognitive or intra- and interpersonal] of the analyst and the patient.
>
> (p. 511; see also Wegner, 1988, 1992, 2011, 2012, 2014b)

All opening scenes collated from initial psychoanalytic interviews were systematically discussed by a fixed group, with hypotheses being derived on the patient's central psychodynamics. In a second step, the relevance of these hypotheses was gauged by external assessors. In summary, the study found evidence that "the opening scene has significant diagnostic importance" (Wegner, 2014a, p. 511); an incidental finding was that the "psychoanalytic method, at least the ability to observe and verbalize clinically and diagnostically relevant data, is teachable and learnable" (Wegner & Henseler, 1991, p. 221, own translation). These two findings provided empirical support for the further development of a group-based method using reduced or concentrated clinical material (the opening scene of a session) that was to be used for the training and continuing professional development of psychoanalysts. The research findings also indicated that the discussion of the material emerging from the FCG should be steered towards the inner reality, the meaning of the parties' inner-psychic processes, and the attendant emotional outcomes. This places a focus on the perception and identification of central affects that accompany and favourably support the search for a "transformational object" (Sklar et al., 2020).

The findings of Morgenthaler and Wegner, by reducing the clinical material presented for discussion, have made two things possible: the condensed presentation and development of the emotional content of the current treatment situation and the expansion to include all the aspects that can develop an effect under, behind, and beside the superficial meaning and diversify the transference and countertransference processes.

Having retraced the developmental steps leading to FCG, we now turn to how the groups work in practice.

The Method of Free Clinical Groups (FCG)

FCG were first offered at the annual conference of the European Psychoanalytical Federation (EPF) in London in 2010 while Peter Wegner was serving as president and Jonathan Sklar as vice-president. Additionally, FCG were run at the 46th IPAC in Chicago, USA, in 2009, and at the 28th Latin American Psychoanalytic Congress (FEPAL) in Bogotá, Colombia, in 2010.

The choice of name "Free Clinical Groups" is intended to signal that the method does not ascribe to a particular theoretical school of psychoanalysis, but that it brings general Freudian ideas to the fore: the meaning of the unconscious, the method of free association, and free-floating or evenly suspended attention.

FCG sessions proceed as follows: an analyst presents clinical material from a clinical session or an initial interview up until the point of the first verbal intervention, without reporting that intervention and without giving any further explanations. The analyst does not yet describe how the session continued or answer any of the comprehension questions that are often posed but remains silent during the following discussion.

The participants then discuss their ideas about the *inner reality* of the analysand, the analyst, and the relationship manifesting between the two. Finally, the participants attempt to construct one or several interventions that could have been delivered in the place of the intervention made by the presenting analyst. Once there is mutual agreement that these steps have been concluded, the analyst is asked to report their own intervention and once that has been discussed, to recount how the session continued. Following a further round of discussion, the presenting analyst reports on the course of treatment and on the patient's biographical background, which can then be discussed. This second step in the FCG method allows the outcomes of the first step to be validated through the provision of biographical data and information on the course of the analysis itself.

The moderators of the group process are experienced colleagues, qualified in the field of psychoanalysis. Their task is to ensure that the group complies with the rules within a psychoanalytic framework: to acknowledge all contributions to the discussion, understanding them from a psychoanalytic perspective, holding them in memory, and drawing connections between them. They thus serve an important function, not only in observing and accompanying the group process, but also in mediating between the group and the presenting analyst.

FCGs thus differ from Balint Groups and other methods of supervision in two decisive ways: first, the group participants are not informed about the case history or treatment of the patient/analysand; the only background information given is age and gender. Second, after the material has been presented and a first "free" discussion has taken place, all participants are asked to formulate a possible interpretation. This difference is important, because it prevents know–it–all–ism on the part of the presenter; instead, participants can or must identify with the presenter's problem. This fundamentally changes the tone of the group: presenter and participants suddenly find themselves "in the same boat."

Beyond functioning as a form of continuing professional development, use of the method has led to the development of new techniques for the assessment of the group discussions, which are recorded and then transcribed. The transcripts are then analyzed at the "micro-process" level within the moderator group and another layer of interpretation added – thus, a new research perspective has been developed. The volume *Mikroprozesse psychoanalytischen Arbeitens* (Danckwardt et al., 2014) charts the FCG method's development from a training tool to a research tool, for example, for analytic process research. The prism effect not only makes unconscious desires and defence mechanisms more visible, it also reveals process identifications, as reactions to the latent processes of exchange in the analytic dyad (see Dankwardt, 2014, pp. 171–172). Any point in a treatment process (e.g., initial interview, short- or long-term treatment, end of treatment) can have particular characteristics that are shaped by the parties involved. The number and diversity of ideas voiced in the group discussions also reflect – unconsciously, pre-consciously, and consciously – these points in the process; they implicitly construct a developmental model of relational experiences and/or their fixations. Elementary components of a lifelong search for a "transformational object" (see, e.g., Bollas, 1992, pp. 11ff.) also emerge from the process, as is generally also assumed to happen in self-awareness processes.

A first comparative study comparing the classic dual "examination situation" in an analytical psychotherapy with the work of FCG was published in 2018 by Peter Wegner (part 1) and by Peter Wegner and Claudia Thußbas (part 2) with the title "Fine-Grained Mental Substances in the Psychoanalytic Situation" ("Feinkörnige Strömungen seelischer Substanzen in der Psychoanalytischen Situation"). Informed by the results of this comparative study, we now posit that the "fine-grained flows" or "micro-processes" between the analytic dyad identified in group discussion describe four elements in the process of the psychoanalytic situation. On one dimension, two of these elements relate to processes within the psychoanalytic situation ("synchronization" and "break") and two to processes between sessions ("self-efficacy" and "recombining pathological self-organization"). On another dimension, two of the elements represent progressive tendencies striving for change ("synchronization" and "self-efficacy") and two indicate retention and compulsive repetition ("break" and "recombining pathological self-organization"). Note that the concepts of progression and retention are solely intended to indicate a direction and do not imply any judgment on the value, necessity, or meaning of the element in question. A break can prove to be just as lifesaving as a synchronization (see also Wegner & Thußbas, 2018, p. 119).

The concept of "fine-grained mental substances in the psychoanalytic situation" (Wegner, 2018) makes the concept of "micro-processes" more precise by supplementing it with a psychosomatic or somatic dimension. The term "psychoanalytic situation" comes from Leo Stone (1061/1973), who used it to conceptualize the doctor–patient relationship and the specific nature of the psychoanalytic setting (Wegner, 2018, p. 175). The four micro-processes were identified in detailed investigations of the discussions of various groups using the FCG method.

"Synchronization" refers to an aspect of the psychoanalytic situation – a falling into step or shared rhythm of patient and analyst. "Synchronization" can, however, merely reflect the desire for a shared rhythm, for example, when a patient has lost the ability to feel the rhythm of their psychic functioning through pathological processes. The ability to achieve synchronization within a patient–analyst situation such as an initial interview can be a significant factor in embarking on a course of psychoanalytic treatment. Synchronization processes have been the subject of a variety of empirical investigations in experimental psychology, especially biological and social psychology, over a period of decades (e.g., McClintock, 1971). To date, these studies have not led to a systematic theory of synchronization processes, but they do suggest the existence of physical and mental structures that strive for synchronization (in the manner of secondary drives) and that can operate over different time frames. In this respect, synchronization processes can be understood as an evolutionary achievement of humans that also play a significant role in the psychoanalytic situation, whether initially in the short term and/or in the longer term (Wegner, 2014b, p. 130).

"Self-efficacy" and "recombining pathological self-organization" refer primarily to life outside or between psychoanalytic sessions, but also relate to the individual sessions themselves. "Self-efficacy" describes an attitude, ability, and self-management technique that makes it psychologically possible for the patient to counteract a pathological tendency (e.g., repetition compulsion) or an unconscious conflict and, as a result, to achieve greater stability. This dimension may be an inherent capacity of the patient from the outset. However, it can also develop to varying degrees over the psychoanalytic process (Wegner, 2018, p. 176). Like "self-efficacy," "recombining pathological self-organization" takes effect primarily outside psychoanalytic sessions and can be assumed to be inherent in the patient to a certain degree. In contrast to "self-efficacy," however, it can counteract successful psychoanalytic work (e.g., in the form of a negative therapeutic reaction), and it may also be a response to the fear of loss in psychoanalytic therapy (e.g., in the case of separation after a psychoanalytic session and the threat of a gap before the next session), which the patient may or may not be able to tolerate. This relapse, regression, defensive mechanism, or denial of reality recombines, among other things, instinctive impulses, recurrent symptoms, micropsychotic episodes, and somatic or psychosomatic reactions, unconsciously relating them to the past (forgotten) or longed-for (urgently awaited) psychoanalytic experience, and transporting them more or less strongly back to the ongoing process of transference and countertransference or urgent unconscious instinctive drives. Freud (e.g., 1908/1959, p. 161) attributed corresponding processes a "proliferate" quality and had mental and physical processes (fantasies and drives) in mind.

The final element, "break," emerged from the discussions of the "Berlin Seminar" (Wegner & Thußbas, 2018). Like other terms such as "annul," "negate," "deregulate," "counteract," "non-simultaneity," "overwhelm and dominate," "no resonance" (Joseph, 1993), "attacks on linking" (Bion, 1959), or "grey noise," the term "break" refers to tendencies that counteract a positive development, interrupt the relationship between patient and analyst, or destroy it for very different reasons. The discussion and further analysis of the Berlin Seminar on a patient whom we called Mr. S. led to the idea that this patient needs enough time and an analyst who allows himself to be both destroyed and loved without taking revenge (Freud, 1955/1909; Lear, 2002; Ogden, 2016; Winnicott, 1969). Here, the central "fine-grained flow" is the "break" that helps the patient to defend himself against the fear of a "breakdown" (Winnicott, 1969). A "psychosomatic collusion" (Winnicott, 1974) may also be part of what is happening in Mr. S.'s case (Wegner & Thußbas, 2018, p. 119).

These processes unfold in FCG by the same routes as described by Loch. The multiplicity of identifications and reaction formations and the variety of ideas expressed bring these processes to the group's consciousness or to the proximity of consciousness. Through its detailed psychoanalytic work at the micro-level, the group seeks to construct options of intervention or interpretation that – it is hoped – reflect an accurate understanding of the patient's psychic reality, support its development, and are better able to trigger potential transformations. It is precisely in the countless details of reflection, in transference and countertransference identifications, and in transference and countertransference reaction formations that forms of psychoanalytic work emerge in which the two participating parties necessarily become attuned to each other.

The parties must also adapt to each other with respect to time, that is, to synchronize with each other. The FCG method thus facilitates predictions not only about resources and causalities, but also on the temporal dimension – not least, predictions about the likely reasons for the chosen frequency of sessions. This essentially opens an entirely new perspective for addressing questions on the indications for different frequencies of psychoanalytic treatment (Danckwardt et al., 2014, pp. 10–11; Wegner, 2014b, pp. 128–130).

Example of a Group Discussion Using the Options of Interpretation Method: Session 103 With Mr. S. in the "Berlin Seminar"

Introduction

To illustrate the workings of FCG, we now present an example of a group discussion that followed the options of interpretation method described earlier. The clinical material for the discussion came from the 103rd session with Mr. S., a patient aged about 50 (Wegner, 2018). Peter Wegner presented the session long after the course of treatment had finished in what we called the Berlin Seminar. The participants were 11 colleagues from the Berlin Psychoanalytical Institute (Karl Abraham Institute). The seminar was moderated by Dorothee von Tippelskirch-Eissing. Claudia Thußbas acted as a passive group observer. Both have been serving as moderators of FCG at the EPF annual conferences for years.

Mr. S.'s 103rd session was presented to the group in the following way: to begin, the analyst presented the start of the session up to his first intervention, which he did not report. The group worked on this material in a first round of discussion lasting almost an hour. The presenting analyst did not participate in the discussion. The second round of discussion, which took another half hour, focused on further material from the session, namely, from the first intervention until shortly before the third intervention. We chose this segment because the second intervention in the session was a repetition of the first one, whereas the third intervention took up a new central theme. Finally, the presenting analyst described the end of the session, and gave some important biographical information and details on the course of the treatment.

Opening Material From Mr. S.'s 103rd Session

First, the moderator spoke some words of welcome and gave a short introduction to the structure of the group session and the FGC method; the clinical session was then introduced. The beginning of the session presented to the participants for the first round of discussion was as follows:

A: *Male patient, aged about 50. I have barely opened the door when he darts away from one of the pictures in the corridor, in which he had been immersed, and hurtles towards me. His mouth opens like a snapper, the keys on his keyring clatter loudly. Mr. S. begins talking quickly, as if he were giving a speech under time pressure. I pretend to listen to him, but internally I move away even though I realize: He's telling me something important.*

S: After our last session, where it was all about my difficulties deciding on anything, I did something unusual that I hadn't done for a long time. When I got back, I didn't feel like writing. I wanted to deliberately kill time playing a computer game. So . . . I decided . . . I'm going to make a conscious decision to do that now. And then I got a game out: Civilization. An ancient classic. My old version didn't run anymore, so I had to download the new version first. Then I played it for a few hours . . . quite a long time . . . until 4 this morning. And then I stopped because I thought if I carried on, our session today wasn't going to happen. . . .

I have to admit, it was as if I'd been up drinking all night. Like a hangover, with a headache . . . . even though I didn't have anything to drink. The point is, I don't even think it's a bad thing. Like a child who desperately wants to puff on cigarettes. . . . It was also a kind of trip back in time for me . . . back to the time with Stephanie. I often did it back then . . . I don't regret it . . . I just wanted to experience that feeling again. It's just burning time and there's nothing left. . . .

A: *He repeats himself again and again. I try to get a word in edgeways. . . . I notice that I'm in danger of drifting away . . . then I say . . .*

Course of the Group Discussion

The participants in the Berlin Seminar plunged straight into the material. The first contributions to the discussion related to drifting away, whether in the context of the nonverbal opening scene where the patient seemed to have drifted away while looking at the pictures, or in the form of observations about their own behaviour while listening to the presentation. For example, participant 8 noted that she had problems focusing on the material while listening. These comments suggest that even while they were first tuning into the clinical material, some participants were already receptive to the countertransference responses of the presenting analyst and were beginning to identify with them.

After about 15 to 20 minutes of discussion, the group entered an almost manic state of activity. Participants picked up on aspects of the opening scene, such as the clattering of the patient's keys, condensing them to concepts such as "latchkey child," which were then taken up by several further participants, feeding into their own associations and ideas, and being passed on to other participants. The passive group observer experienced this part of the discussion as a kind of whirlwind, a flurry of associations, each voiced at speed, but at the same time seeming to circle around an unspoken stillness or inertia. At this point, the group seems to have strongly identified with the patient's intellectualizing pseudo-creativity, which was clearly apparent in later parts of the session. This shows the psychical *resonance effect* of the group mentioned earlier, a reflection within the group of the psychodynamic condition of sickness.

The whirlwind was finally halted by a comment from participant 4, who suddenly ventured something new. She reminded the rest of the group that the patient had also achieved something – he had been able to stop gaming. And it was this break that had allowed him to come to the session. This comment not only introduced new content to the discussion, but it also put a stop to the group's pseudo-activity. Now the group could move on to grasping the patient's inner object world in a totally new way. For the first time, the participants also named affects that they inferred in the patient, or that they experienced directly: they spoke of rage and guilt, but also of sorrow and desolation. The observations associated were increasingly sensory in nature, leaving the level of object relations.

Finally, the group showed a psychosomatic response. Participant 3 was the first to notice that she had begun to feel cold. Almost collectively, many participants registered at this point in the discussion that they had, without realizing, begun to feel terribly cold. This both surprising and unpleasant physical condition in the group ultimately enabled the participants to understand the patient's emotional distress even better. The group became able to feel, recognize, and comprehend the patient's fragile object relations, brittle perception of reality, and catastrophically hate-filled self-relations. With the moderator's support, the participants' comments were translated into options of interpretation that related to loneliness, having to wait, and the difficulty of remaining in contact with oneself and with the analyst.

Moreover, a comment made by participant 3, which related to the analyst's capacity to get through to the patient, offered a further option of interpretation, the effect of which did not fully come to bear until the subsequent group discussion. She said:

> I wonder with this patient whether, when one formulates a feeling, it's more or less nonsense for the patient. . . . And that it could be a different matter for physical sensations, like feeling cold . . . where he'd have the feeling of being understood.
> (Wegner & Thußbas, 2018, p. 105, own translation)

In feeling cold and reflecting on that condition, the members of the Berlin Seminar thus sensed the "break" that helped the patient to ward off the fear of a breakdown and, specifically, to come to the session, by way of psychosomatic collusion (see Winnicott, 1974). Mr. S. and his analyst had not yet had this experience at the respective point in the treatment. The group thus intuitively developed a concept that was inherent in the unconscious movements of transference and countertransference, but that had not yet been thought in the treatment.

This concept was to be validated by clinical material from later in the treatment. For example, a passage from an unpublished novel that Mr. S. had not yet written at the time of the 103rd session demonstrates that Mr. S. was himself occupied with feeling cold in a psychologically meaningful way. In the words of the book's protagonist (our translation): "The sunny cold breaks into his inner space, his innermost recesses. He wants to sleep. He can smell it, the cold."

The clinical working group in our example thus worked together using the method of options of interpretation and, after overcoming a phase of manic activity, achieved true creativity. Participant 3's comment, which was not only sensitively received, but stayed with the group throughout, enabled the participants to formulate new thoughts on the treatment. By the end of the discussion, the group had grasped the relevance of the coldness of the patient's earlier environment, of his primary reference persons, as well as his own inner coldness, and was able to offer an interpretation of it.

Closing Thoughts on the Future Development of the FCG Method

The aim of working together in a group is to deepen the understanding of the analyst–patient relationship, which in turn makes it possible to reflect on a specific therapeutic intervention. In our diverse experience, the strengths of this form of group work can be attributed to two main features: the participants' reflection on the case presented is not primarily an intellectual endeavour; rather, it often is the result of a collective recognition and processing of a central affect in the treatment. In the example presented here, it was only when one participant's comment put a stop to the group's manic burst of activity that it was at all possible to work on the affects, which – in the segment of the session presented – had seemed to be frozen. It was only through the group's psychosomatic response – feeling cold – that the patient's harsh and narcissistic affect-lessness became apparent to the group, could be "thawed out" in joint work, and then flowed into options of interpretation. This group process is an example of successful clinical practice in which an affect that was frozen during the session itself was experienced by the group and could even, to some extent, be processed.

The FCG method sidesteps any school-specific intellectualization of the case, not only by rendering the unconscious identifications and defences in the treatment visible but also, and above all, by rendering them flexible. As shown earlier, group members can identify by turns with the presenting analyst, the patient, and the analytic process over the course of the group session. By working through both sides, the group can think its way to a new conceptualization.

Loch notes that Balint groups will fail to achieve their aims if they turn into self-awareness groups or proceed in the style of psychotherapeutic supervision sessions. These same risks also apply to our groups. But this is where the work of the moderators comes in. If the moderators are able to tolerate the flexibilization of unconscious dynamics in the group and to prompt the group members and the presenter to ask who is speaking to whom at the unconscious level, the method affords all participants a deep clinical experience with the unconscious processes of the patient whose case is presented. Moreover, a space emerges in which they can work through psychodynamic affects that have not yet been considered.

We have now applied the FCG method and studied its effects in diverse clinical contexts. For example, master's students in the Leadership and Counselling course at the International Psychoanalytic University Berlin are supervised using the method. Clinical working groups with psychoanalysts in training have also worked with it successfully. Finally, clinical working groups that have already been working together for some time also seem to be able to benefit from the introduction of the method, as demonstrated by examples such as a clinical working group of colleagues in the United States who used the method together with German colleagues for the first time. As a discourse-oriented method that aims to facilitate mutual understanding between subjects, this psychoanalytic method is particularly well suited to facilitating a clinical understanding between different psychoanalytical schools and traditions. The group is interested not only in a psychoanalytic process but also, and primarily, in arriving at possible interpretations.

In this context, the method not only enhanced the participants' clinical work, but also, by laying bare group dynamics, afforded them insights into the various identities of the participants and the internal conflict dynamics that manifest in treatments. Initially unaware of the patient's history, the group may – in the absence of that knowledge – be unconsciously more attuned to the possible rhythms of affect. In traditional clinical presentations, where background information is provided, the group can understand the material intellectually but not necessarily emotionally. This is perhaps a major difference from the FCG approach presented here, where participants are somewhat distanced from the material, especially from the patient's early childhood environment, and instead the intensity of affect is transmitted to the group.

Despite or perhaps because of the direct emotionality of this form of group work, it seems to nourish participants' passion for psychoanalytic work. An element of Loch's personality and of his clinical work is conveyed through the method, making him experienceable, even after his death.

Considering the group dynamics that emerge when colleagues join forces to work on a clinical case is far from a new concept in the field of psychoanalysis. Yet although the process is often experienced as exceptionally fruitful, it is a perspective that often seems to be lost in clinical supervisory practice.

Notes

1 We are particularly grateful to the following regular moderators: Ursula Burkert (German Association), Milagros Cid Sanz (Madrid Association), Henrik Enckell (Finnish Psychoanalytical Society), Patrick Miller (Paris Society), Denny Panitz (Hellenic Society), Manuela Utrilla Robles (Madrid Association), Jonathan Sklar (British Society), Claudia Thußbas (German Association), Dorothee von Tippelskirch-Eissing (German Association), Christine Wegner (German Association), Peter Wegner (German Association), and Marja Wille-Buurman (Dutch Society).
2 Translation of this sentence from Hinz (2008, p. 124).
3 At this conference, Wolfgang Loch and Gemma Jappe led a clinical seminar entitled "Deutungs-Optionen? Überlegungen zur Frage der Interpretationsebenen anhand eines Stundenprotokolls" (Loch & Jappe, 1990), which laid the methodological groundwork for the later Achalm Seminars. It also paved the way for a specific method of supervision or intervision for psychoanalytic training in the stricter sense or for the continuing professional development of psychoanalysts in clinical practice, which we then later developed further in the context of FCG.

Bibliography

Balint, M. (1964). *The doctor, his patient and the illness.* Pitman Medical Publishing.

Bion, W. R. (1959). Attacks on linking. *International Journal of Psychoanalysis, 40,* 308–315.

Bollas, C. (1992). *Being a character: Psychoanalysis and self experience.* Hill & Wang.

Dankwardt, J. F. (2014). Einige Prozesselemente psychoanalytischen Arbeitens [Some process elements of psychoanalytic work]. In J. F.

Danckwardt, G. Schmithüsen, & P. Wegner (Eds.), *Mikroprozesse psychoanalytischen Arbeitens* (pp. 167–187). Brandes & Apsel.

Danckwardt, J. F., Schmithüsen, G., & Wegner, P. (2014). *Mikroprozesse psychoanalytischen Arbeitens [Microprocesses of psychoanalytic work]*. Brandes & Apsel.

Freud, S. (1955). Notes upon a case of obsessional neurosis. In J. Strachey (Ed. & Trans.), *The standard edition of the complete psychological works of Sigmund Freud* (Vol. 10, pp. 153–249). Hogarth Press. (Original work published 1909).

Freud, S. (1959). Hysterical phantasies and their relation to bisexuality. In J. Strachey (Ed. & Trans.), *The standard edition of the complete psychological works of Sigmund Freud* (Vol. 9, pp. 159–166). Hogarth Press. (Original work published 1908).

Haas, J.-P. (1995). Zur Psychodynamik der Unechtheit [On the psychodynamics of inauthenticity]. In J.-P. Haas, & G. Jappe (Eds.), *Deutungs-Optionen. Für Wolfgang Loch* (pp. 151–188). Edition Discord.

Hinz, H. (2008). Some reflections on the problem of comparison and difference in the light of doubts and enthusiasm. In D. Tuckett (Ed.), *Psychoanalysis comparable and incomparable: The evolution of the method to describe and compare psychoanalytic approaches* (pp. 95–131). Routledge.

Joseph, B. (1993). Ein Faktor, der psychischer Veränderung entgegenwirkt: Keine Resonanz [A factor militating against psychic change: Non-Resonance]. *Psyche – Z Psychoanal, 47*, 997–1012.

Lear, J. (2002). Jumping from the couch. *International Journal of Psychoanalysis, 83* (3), 583–595.

Loch, W. (1966). Studien zur Dynamik, Genese und Therapie der frühen Objektbeziehungen. Michael Balints Beitrag zur Theorie der frühen Objektbeziehungen [Studies on the dynamics, genesis and therapy of early object relations. Michael Balint's contribution to the theory of early object relations]. *Psyche – Z Psychoanal, 20*, 881–903.

Loch, W. (1972). Psychotherapeutische Behandlung psychosomatischer Erkrankungen [Psychotherapeutic treatment of psychosomatic illnesses]. In W. Loch (Ed.), *Zur Theorie, Technik und Therapie der Psychoanalyse* (pp. 269–282). S. Fischer.

Loch, W. (1992). Mein Weg zur Psychoanalyse. Über das Zusammenwirken familiärer, gesellschaftlicher und individueller Faktoren [My way to psychoanalysis. On the interaction of family, social and individual factors]. In L. M. Herrmanns (Ed.), *Psychoanalyse in Selbstdarstellungen I* (pp. 203–236). Edition Discord.

Loch, W. (1995). *Theorie und Praxis von Balint-Gruppen [Theory and practice of Balint groups]*. Edition Discord.

Loch, W., & Jappe, G. (1990). Deutungs-Optionen? Überlegungen zur Frage der Interpretationsebenen anhand eines Stundenprotokolls [Options of interpretation? Reflections on the question of levels of interpretation based on a session protocol]. In J. Gutwinski-Jeggle, & P. Wegner (Eds.), *Erleben und Deutung. Ästhetik und Ratio* (pp. 150–158). DER-Congress.

McClintock, M. (1971). Menstrual synchrony and suppression. *Nature, 229*, 244–245.

Morgenthaler, F. (1986). *Der Traum. Fragmente zur Theorie und Technik der Traumdeutung [The dream: Fragments on the theory and technique of dream interpretation]*. Edition Qumran im Campus Verlag.

Ogden, T. H. (2016). Destruction reconceived: On Winnicott's "The use of an object and relating through identifications." *International Journal of Psychoanalysis, 97* (5), 1243–1262.

Sklar, J. (2017). *Balint matters: Psychosomatics and the art of assessment*. Karnac.

Sklar, J., Thußbas, C., & Wegner, P. (2020). Michael Balint, Wolfgang Loch und die Weiterentwicklung der Methode der "Freien klinischen Gruppen" [Michael Balint, Wolfgang Loch, and the Development of the "Free Clinical Groups Method"]. *Luzifer-Amor, 66*, 36–54.

Wegner, P. (1988). *Die Bedeutung der Anfangsszene im psychoanalytischen Erstinterview [The importance of the opening scene in the initial psychoanalytical interview]*. [Doctoral dissertation]. Universität Tübingen.

Wegner, P., & Henseler, H. (1991). Die Anfangsszene im Prisma einer Analytikergruppe [The opening scene in the prism of a group of psychoanalysts]. *Forum Psychoanal, 7* (3), 214–224.

Wegner, P. (1992). Zur Bedeutung der Gegenübertragung im psychoanalytischen Erstinterview [The opening scene and the importance of the countertransference in the initial psychoanalytic interview]. *Psyche – Z Psychoanal, 3* (46), 286–307.

Wegner, P. (2011). The opening scene and the importance of the countertransference in the initial psychoanalytic interview. In B. Reith, S. Lagerlöf, P. Crick, M. Møller, & E. Skale (Eds.), *Initiating psychoanalysis: Perspectives* (pp. 226–242). Routledge.

Wegner, P. (2012). Process-orientated psychoanalytical work in the first interview and the importance of the opening scene. *Psychoanalysis in Europe: Bulletin, 66*, 23–45.

Wegner, P. (2014a). Process-orientated psychoanalytical work in initial interviews and the importance of the opening scene. *International Journal of Psychoanalysis, 95* (3), 505–523.

Wegner, P. (2014b). Untersuchung eines Erstinterviews. Frau Z. [Study on an initial interview: Mrs. Z.]. In J. F. Danckwardt, G. Schmithüsen,

& P. Wegner (Eds.), *Mikroprozesse psychoanalytischen Arbeitens* (pp. 113–134). Brandes & Apsel.

Wegner, P. (2018). Feinkörnige Strömungen seelischer Substanzen in der psychoanalytischen Situation (Teil 1) [Fine-grained mental substances in the psychoanalytic situation: Part 1]. *JB Psychoanal*, *76*, 165–192.

Wegner, P., & Thußbas, C. (2018). Feinkörnige Strömungen seelischer Substanzen in der psychoanalytischen Situation (Teil 2) [Fine-grained mental substances in the psychoanalytic situation: Part 2]. *JB Psychoanal*, *77*, 97–122.

Winnicott, D. W. (1969). The use of an object and relating through identifications. *International Journal of Psychoanalysis*, *50* (4), 711–716.

Winnicott, D. W. (1974). Fear of breakdown. *International Review of Psychoanalysis*, *1*, 103–107.

Translated from German by Susannah Goss

9

WORKING PARTY ON PSYCHOSOMATICS – EPF

"A Journey of Exploration" (2012–2020)

Marina Perris-Myttas, with the participation of
Bérengère de Senarclens, Jacques Press, and Christian Seulin

How might a sustained open dialogue among nine psychoanalysts from six different European countries working from a variety of psychoanalytic perspectives enlarge and complicate understandings of effective clinical engagement with psychosomatic patients? This chapter offers readers a window into our working group's processes, not to suggest a theory of psychosomatics, but rather to raise questions, propose hypotheses, and advance lines of investigation related to the psychosomatic condition.

Introduction

In this chapter, we will present the work of our EPF Working Party on Psychosomatics. We aim to reflect upon the journey we travelled, and on how, in writing a book together, we became observers of our own work. This endeavor, complex, nuanced, and multifaceted as it was, offered us enriching and rewarding challenges.

The Method

Our "core group"[1] is made of nine psychoanalysts coming from six different European countries, from diverse psychoanalytic traditions, different theoretical approaches, and clinical practices. Our

DOI: 10.4324/9781032656311-9

driving force was a wish to exchange, discuss, and explore these various perspectives while working with psychosomatic patients. Our first decision was to start this venture by exchanges involving our clinical work with somatic patients.

Our group met two or three weekends each year since 2012. On the first day of these gatherings, we focused on case presentations, offered by one of us to the group. This gave us the opportunity to observe our ways of working and our technical and theoretical approaches. In these case presentations, we quickly realized the importance of electing one of us to play the role of a "silent observer" whose task was to trace implicit theoretical hypotheses that infiltrated the clinical work presented. This method allowed us to discern and debate our divergences, a process which enabled us to arrive at specific *ideas* with regard to understanding psychosomatic patients. Our aim was not to suggest a theory of psychosomatics, nor did we intend to develop one. Essentially, we tried to raise questions, to propose hypotheses, and to advance further lines of investigation related to the psychosomatic condition.

Starting our work from the analysis of clinic material gave rise to our working structure. This structure consisted of three components: the weekend meetings of the core group itself – the heart of the structure; the full day clinical workshops that took place at the annual EPF congresses; and the panel on psychosomatics that became a feature of these yearly international meetings. These events were led by us, members of the core group.

These three components and the various clinical and theoretical discussions that emerged from them form the overall configuration that allowed us to advance our hypotheses on the psychosomatic condition. At the same time, this structure proved to be not only a safe carrier of the group's intermittent conflictual processes and dynamics, but also became a safe vehicle for us to collectively produce our book *Experiencing the Body: A Psychoanalytic Dialogue in Psychosomatics*. The book, as such, reflects our way of functioning, our "methodology."

The chapter here presented focuses first and foremost on seizing the complexity of what came to be perceived as the two layers of the functioning of the group. The first layer pertains to our collective wish to remain as near as possible to the experience of the analyst at work through tracing the unfolding of the relationship of the analytic "couple," while aiming at deepening our understanding of the psychic world of our somatic patients. The second layer refers to our wish to maintain a constant observation and self-reflection regarding our group dynamics. We also remained attentive to the parallel processes between the two layers.

This chapter is made of three parts. The first one develops further the presentation of our way of working together. The second part is the exposition of an actual panel that took place at the EPF conference in Warsaw (2018). The third part is a brief account of the themes we chose to elaborate in our book, the presentation of some important themes we agreed on. We then proceed to suggest some "new lines," thoughts and explorations, for further investigation in psychosomatics, which we see emerging from our work over the last seven years.

The Core Group

We shall start by looking at the core group which is the Working Party's initial structure: the place from which our enterprise evolved, a "work group" in Bion's (1961) terms (Shields, 2016). As already said, we were nine psychoanalysts interested in psychosomatics and working with physically ill patients. The quest of the group was to deepen and *open up* the psychoanalytic understanding of the psychosomatic condition. The backbone of our work has been our psychoanalytic practice. Presenting clinical cases to each other furnished the material needed for our endeavor. This process was productive.

As J. Press (2019) describes, we each had to confront unfamiliar ways of thinking and tolerate differences between us. But we also had to confront and make explicit what was often implicit in our own way of thinking and thereby become more aware of it. Moreover, we quickly realized that while we encountered divergences in our understanding of the material and in our styles of intervention, we were nonetheless able to find common ground. In the discussions of the clinical cases, we focused on the quality of the analyst's listening, and on the movements of transference and countertransference.

As we progressed, the question of the specificity of psychosomatics became central and we came to a working understanding that the subject matter of the field of psychosomatics is concerned with the exploration and understanding of the psychic organization and functioning, as well as the circumstances – internal and external – that are likely to destabilize the individual's psychosomatic balance, leading to an eruption of somatic symptoms whose economic and, at times, symbolic value is crucial for our work.

In addition, psychosomatics is concerned with the following question: how might the work of analysis contribute to the mitigation of the processes of somatization, and from there, how might the patient be helped to move (or to return) to a psychosomatic equilibrium, an equilibrium which, when things are going well, is to be found (in the main), under the auspices of *Eros* – the life drive.

A few questions remain: what about the group dynamics? How do these relate to our elaboration of the psychoanalytic work with patients at the time of physical illness?

Indeed, over time we became increasingly aware of the value that the study of group processes could bring to our investigations. So we invested ourselves in observing these processes. This investment permeated our structure as a whole and took on different articulations in its different components.

First, our commitments with regard to the core group: within this group we took care, albeit implicitly, to recognize and register the group dynamics as they emerged. Through a tacit agreement, we steadily aimed at containing the inevitable areas of conflict. In relation to this stance, and with the benefit of hindsight, the following question comes to mind. Can we think of this mode of dealing with the conflict – by containing it – as an implication of a parallel process that reflects the elemental necessity of containment in our clinical work with physically ill patients? The kind of work, which is so rooted in and dependent upon – we repeatedly found – the analyst's readiness to hold the excessive affective movements, is often the result of trauma, as well as the ensuing unrepresented states of mind that are consistently present in patients who suffer from physical illness (Marty, 1958; Aisenstein, 2007; Miller, 2018). In other words, we came to wonder whether the route we took – by and large dealing with the intensities and conflictual group dynamics by containment – proceeded from the dynamics present in the analytic work with the physically ill patient, as reflected in the workings of the group through parallel processes.

A second complementary and rather heuristic question arises at this point: did our actual way of working with somatic patients, as it is in our stance of containing excessive intensities, make us particularly sensitive to both the dynamics in our group and to the vital need for the intense affects to be contained in order for our work to be facilitated and to progress?

Let us now turn to the next components of our structure and focus on what we came to perceive as the prevailing stance in our work, the constant observation and reflection on our experiences and unfolding processes.

The Clinical Workshops at European Psychoanalytic Federation Conference

In these clinical workshops, group dynamics were explicitly explored. We ran two simultaneous groups which took place in the EPF pre-conference time. The presenters in these workshops were psychoanalysts from different countries and psychoanalytic societies. They brought for discussion clinical material from their work with somatically ill patients. Each group was regulated by three of four members of the core group, with one of them having the role of "silent observer." While the clinical exploration remained the aim of the workshop, we also came to witness how the dynamics presented in the material were reflected in the dynamics of the group. Working with the clinical material presented brought to the fore the centrality of the movements of the transference/countertransference in working with the economic fragility of physically ill patients. The often powerful presence of these movements repeatedly re-emerged in the dynamics of the clinical workshop. The silent observer was tasked with locating these dynamics. When possible, he offered thoughts regarding the parallel processes that ran through the patient's psychosomatic struggle, the movements of the transference/countertransference, and the observed dynamics in the workshop. These observations were then offered to the group for exploration.

At the end of the two workshops, the core group carries out a reflective meeting to further elaborate on the work. A further vantage point (a meta-third position) emerges in this meeting. Notwithstanding the density and at times confusion built into these elaborations, we have often been astounded by the rich insights that they have afforded us. Indeed, with time, the experiences in the clinical workshops found expression both in transforming the structure of the Panel on Psychosomatics, and in the very making of the book.

Panel on Psychosomatics

The Panel on Psychosomatics took place every year at the EPF annual conference. Two points about these panels: first, the transformation that they underwent, and second, the contribution of the panels' structure in shaping the form of the book.

The panel's initial form consisted of three parallel papers on the theme of each conference presented by three members of the core group. With time, however, by taking our lead from the experiences in the clinical workshops and from the developing dialogue within the core group, the arrangement of our annual panel transformed. In the new form we still have three panelists. But we now have one panelist who presents a clinical paper and two discussants. Our aim is to present the thinking of our group in a form of dialogue that communicates the diverse nuances of our thinking and invites further discussion. This new arrangement has informed the making of our book, that which materialized along the lines of a dialogue.

We shall proceed now to the exposition of the actual panel presented at the EPF conference in Warsaw. In doing so, we hope to give an in-depth view of our way of working, firmly grounded on theoretical and clinical dialogue, of our understanding of psychosomatic patients, and of the demands of the analytic work at times of physical illness.

An Example: Marina Perris[2]

In "Interpretation of Dreams," Freud (1900/1955) invites us to closely observe an infant in the grip of an urgent somatic need, hunger, at a moment of heightened excitation:

> A hungry baby screams or kicks helplessly. . . . A change can only come about if in some way or other an "experience of satisfaction" can be achieved which puts an end to the internal stimulus [(hunger)].
>
> An essential component of this experience of satisfaction is a particular perception (here that of nourishment), the mnemic image of which remains associated thenceforward with the memory trace of the excitation produced by the need.
>
> As a result of the link that has thus been established, next time this need arises a psychical impulse will at once emerge which

will seek to re-cathect the mnemic image of the perception and to re-evoke the perception itself, that is to say, to re-establish the situation of the original satisfaction. An impulse of this kind is what we call a wish; the reappearance of the perception is the fulfilment of the wish.

(p. 565)

This passage succinctly and lucidly brings into focus two critical matters. First, it points to the origins of the psychic in the somatic: from the somatic experience of the infant's suffering from hunger to the baby who gets to the psychic experience of having a wish. Second, in the expression "the original satisfaction," we can recognize, albeit in the light of the rigor of the developments in psychoanalytic theory since 1900, the presence of the object. More specifically, the object in its mediating function, the object who enables the transition from the somatic to the psychic and, in the process, potentiates the constitution of the drive and the establishment of the psychosomatic unity.

Fifteen years later, Freud (1915/1957) elucidates and substantiates this moment of transition in his definition of the drive:

If now we apply ourselves to considering mental life from a biological point of view, a drive (1) appears to us as a concept on the frontier between the mental and the somatic, as the psychical representative of the stimuli originating from within the organism, and reaching the mind as a measure of the demand made upon the mind for work in consequence of its connection with the body.

(p. 121–122)

Freud postulates that the stimuli originate from within the organism. A process is then initiated, and through its unfolding, a demand for work is eventually placed upon the mind. It is in the meeting of this demand that the drive is constituted as the psychic representative of the somatic. think that Andre Green (2010) depicts the onset of this process very eloquently when he describes "the stimuli originating from within the soma" as the "mooring of the somatic" (p. 40). Following Freud, Green sees the soma as always there from the beginning: the soma is the actuality of the organism from which excitation originates. Green, moreover, contends that the somatic excitations initially reach the "first zone of transition,

202

which I consider to be absolutely fundamental, which is the somato-psychic barrier: no one speaks about it, but it is of cardinal importance" (p. 40). In my opinion, following on from this "first zone of transition" during unobstructed development comes the demand upon the mind and the constitution of the drive: somatic excitations meet with perceptions and memory traces; the libidinal body comes into being and the psychic world unfolds. Once at work, these processes mutually foster each other's development.

When considering the origins of psychic life in the soma, the notion of the object partaking as it is in the constitution of the drive is of momentous significance. In Green's (2002) words,

> The concept of the drive is unthinkable without the object. The proof of this is that the object is part of the drive assembly. Furthermore, the object thus conceived always implies an object that is external to this assembly and independent of it at the outset, ensuring functions of survival.
>
> (p. 63)

Further the fate of the unfolding of the psychic development crucially depends on the primary object who, from the very first instance, mediates the transition from the somatic to the psychic. The actuality, the attributes, and the capabilities of the mediating object can obstruct or facilitate this transition, from the somatic excitation to the constitution of the drive, along with the advent of the libidinal body and psychic representations. The function of the "mediating" object as the first object that receives the cathexis of the constituting drive has been focused upon extensively and diversely within the psychoanalytic literature (Ferenczi, 1923; Winnicott, 1992; Klein, 1946; Bion, 1967; Fain, 1971; Laplanche, 1979; Green, 2002).

In the fifties in his book, *Through Paediatrics to Psychoanalysis*, Donald Winnicott brought to the fore the significance of the primary object. Here, he introduced his renowned concept of the "good enough" mother who in the state of "primary maternal preoccupation" allows for the "going on being" of the infant and keeps him safe from intolerable impingements, starting from the time of absolute dependence. For the infant, if all goes well, this "maternal provision" will allow for non–obstructed development first and foremost by securing the "psyche-in-dwelling-in-the-soma," a developmental achievement itself, which, in my opinion, is a very similar process to that of the transition from the somatic to the psychic.

Following Freud, Winnicott turns his attention to the individual's psychosomatic existence. In his words, he invites us to attempt to:

> think of the developing individual, starting in the beginning. Here is a body, and the psyche and the soma are not to be distinguished except according to the direction from which one is looking. One can look at the developing body or at the developing psyche. I suppose psyche means here the imaginative elaboration of somatic parts, feelings and functions, that is of physical aliveness.
>
> (1992, p. 244)

In this same work, Winnicott defines the "mind" as "no more than a special case of the functioning of the psyche–soma" (p. 224). This designation of the mind evokes, in my opinion, Freud's notion of the drive, or rather, the process of the drive's constitution. When the somatic excitation meets with a perception or a memory trace, it becomes a constituent of a drive. The drive then places on the mind a demand for work. Furthermore, albeit outside the scope of this paper, it seems to me that the question can be raised as to whether Winnicott's definition of the psyche as "the imaginative elaboration of somatic parts, feelings and functions" has some affinity with Green's notion of the "moorings of the somatic."

In health, which means in absence of obstruction, the unfolding of the psychic world out of its somatic origins takes its course. When things go wrong, however, we may witness in analysis the reverse movement of the drive: from the psychic to the somatic, which brings in its wake a rupture in the psychic functioning and the eruption of the physical illness.

This rupture gets expressed in the mounting of excess excitation that eventually may reach a point when "the mental apparatus" switches off and "the somatic reaction kicks in, more or less totally, substituting for the psychical reaction" (Smadja, 2005, p. 32). During the analysis of patients who somatize, the analyst might experience in the countertransference the rupture in the psychic functioning caused by the drive's return to its somatic origins.

I will now discuss the period when my patient Liona falls ill during her analysis and the emergence of early maternal trauma experienced, as it was, in the unfolding of the transference and countertransference.

Liona introduced herself by saying, "I am here because I find life impossible." She was in her 30s, had a 3-year-old daughter, and was single. She was dressed in black, and inescapably anxious. She had a long history of somatic illness, mainly gastrointestinal disturbances and eczema, which she had suffered since childhood. In the first consultation she talked about her mother who had Liona in her adolescence. "I was just a child myself," she had told her.

Liona started with three sessions a week, and within a few months, she developed strong enthusiasm for the analytic work, in particular for the setting, and she wanted to come "every day." Indeed, after some time, she embarked in a five-times-a-week analysis, and her anxiety became markedly reduced.

With time, life became less "impossible." She was struggling less in her relationships and stayed free of somatic ailments. There was, however, an ever-present sense of brittleness, which at times immobilized us both.

A few years later, a sense of an infantile traumatic past emerged in the analytic scene, suggested through the deficiency of the coming together of affect and representation. For instance, towards the end of a session in which Liona was extremely anxious about her daughter running a high fever, she said that the night before she was woken up by a "terrible migraine." I said that it seemed to me that her intense worry about her daughter's fever the night before had given her a migraine. I got a sharp and cutting response back: "No, I do not think so." "Anyway," she immediately added in an anxious manner, "I always felt I exist from the neck up. I am here for you to fix my head, this would be enough and I shall be grateful." I was dumbfounded and speechless. Still feeling at a loss after the session, I thought that my intervention failed to facilitate associations and the possibility of making sense and allowing feelings to emerge, other than anxiety. I had the image of disconnected threads and the uneasy feeling of a deep severance between the body and the mind.

I will now focus on the developments that followed the moment my patient had the first awareness that her analysis would, albeit at a future time upon the completion of her PhD thesis, come to an end. This perception of a loss had shaken her still active unconscious

205

belief in our idyllic oneness. At that time, she was experiencing a threat of impending loss, which I sensed she could not find a way to think about. She became increasingly detached both from me and from herself. Her communications became factual, mostly about the logistics of putting together her proposal. She was talking about "life becoming colourless."

I sensed a mounting underlying anxiety while other feelings were disappearing. It seemed that at the prospect of facing the upcoming end of the analysis, under the sway of the transference, split-off early experiences of the traumatic loss in the order of primary narcissism were coming back and being repeated in analysis. Liona started having gastrointestinal problems; she was aching and having severe diarrhea on a daily basis. She was falling ill, following the path of a "somatic regression."

In her adolescence, Liona had suffered from irritable bowel syndrome and her symptoms were coming back. "I check when I go to the toilet to see if the "black color in my feces comes back." I knew that when she was 16 the "black color" was followed by the finding of internal bleeding and horrendously painful episodes of gastric spasms. Liona began to remember all the intrusive tests she had to go through and the pre-cancerous state that was diagnosed. "This is what my doctor thinks goes on now as well," she said. In sharp contrast to her factual and detailed narration, I felt left "in the dark": Liona was no longer talking to me.

I then started to observe myself oscillating in my countertransference. On the one hand, I was anxiously waiting for her, and on the other, I was often close to forgetting her sessions. At that time, and as Liona filled the sessions with her somatic experiences, I started having stomach and intestinal cramps, and I often felt an urge to interrupt the session, as I was feeling sick. My somatic "re-action" was, I thought afterwards, the outcome of a transmission: the excitation which originated in the patient's somatically ill body was being received by her analyst through the somatic reactions in and outside the sessions. During this time, when I was not feeling pain and suffering in my own body, I felt shaken, astounded, worried, and unable to represent to myself whatever it was that was happening to me. An absence of psychic elaboration prevailed in Liona while my own capacity for analytic thinking was also overwhelmed.

One Monday morning, just before the end of her session, Liona said that she had been very anxious about coming to her session that day. She did not want to see me. Drawing on the force of the experience of my physical state the previous week, I said, "You were anxious about what impact you had on me last Friday, you feared I became undone and I would not be here for you today." I felt the fragility of her affective states as I was talking, and I worried about the effect on her tenuous psychosomatic balance. She remained silent, but then I saw her body relaxing on the couch.

She called before her next session, which was on Tuesday evening, to say she was too ill and exhausted to come to see me. Could we speak on the phone? I agreed – which was a questionable response. She told me that most of the bowel investigations came back negative, but that last night she had found a lump, a "mass" in her breast. It was a cyst that she had aspirated immediately. "I am waiting to hear now, the consultant said that there was black blood coming out of the aspiration. This waiting is killing me," she said in a calm voice that impressed me. I was relieved to hear that she was able to wait, albeit with great difficulty. She continued, "will this "mass" be malignant? All these things: the proposal, the interview, my gut problems, now this "mass." I felt relieved at hearing her refer to the proposal; she was making a link between her illness and her sense of impending loss.

I said, "A mass of thoughts and feelings that cannot be fathomed."

Liona responded: "The blackness moved from one place to another."

"And black is for mourning," I replied.

I heard her crying. Eventually she said, "I was not sure that you would still be here today."

The "mass" was not malignant, and after this came a very productive time in the analysis, albeit very painful as her early maternal trauma, which had shown some signs in the past, was becoming increasingly present. She was full of anxiety, but this time the anxiety was not diffused and generalized. On the contrary, it was attached to future prospects that would leave her unprotected. She feared, for instance, that something would "fall apart" in her car and she would find herself "stranded" and maybe attacked in the street on her way to analysis. A fear that we were later able to connect with her fear that I would speak with words that were "cutting and damaging" to her: she would find herself unshielded in the face of this danger. One day she brought the following dream:

> I was in a rather dark room, looking at a little baby girl. There was piercing on her navel, the skin was red, I could not stand it. I was looking at her face, I thought she was numb. I started scream-ing, "who is doing this? She is too little for this." I woke up in terror. When I fell asleep again and the dream came back, I could not get rid of it.

After a pause she added: "I was impressed that I screamed so loud, but glad I did!"

While suggesting some symbolic capacity, the dream also reveals the tenuous quality of Liona's network of representations: it becomes a nightmare and points to primary trauma. Nightmares arise when the dream work is not strong enough to contain the excitation pres-ent in the dreamer, and the sleep then gets disrupted. And yet my patient could not avoid her dream, even as it started turning into a nightmare. As she began falling asleep again, her dream kept com-ing back, kept turning into a nightmare. It kept coming back to deliver its message, I thought.

Working on the dream while living through the rage and terror that the piercing was happening all over again in the here and now of the analytic relationship, we arrived at the idea that the piercing was a repetition, signaling the way her unconscious was taking her and us both back to a time of trauma whose origin led me to think of Ferenczi's (1923) "Confusion of Tongues between the Adult and the Child."

Ferenczi's thoughts are, in my view, reverberated in Winnicott's notion of early maternal impingements which disturb the psyche-in–dwelling–in–the–soma, as well as in Laplanche's (1997) notion of traumatic "untranslatable messages." Dejours (2010) takes Laplanche's idea a step further when he suggests that when the translation of the adult's message fails, the experience remains "recorded as that of a torrent of excitement in the body that leads to a destabilization, indeed a rupture of the ego that is in the process of being formed" (p. 201). As the body's task to translate fails, under the weight of excess of excitation, the ego's integrity is threatened.

In all these theorizations, there is a common thread: the adult's uncontained libidinal unconscious emits untranslatable messages addressed to the infant; the messages become inscribed in the infant's body "as a torrent of excitation" and as such, remain unrepresentable.

Returning to my patient, my understanding is that the mother's holding gestures were experienced as physical violations which were symbolized in the dream by the "piercing": a violent intrusiveness which has permeated the transference and countertransference in different forms and intensities throughout the analysis, including in the somatic transmission. The image of the tender skin of the naval came to my mind: the piercing, the possibility of infection, and the anxious tenacity with which, some years back, she had declared that she could only exist from the neck up.

> I said, "You speak of scarring on the infant's body, there is a fear of an infection that can fester and endanger life."
> "Endanger the life of senses and feelings," she said.

This early scarring was at the root of the disconnection between my patient's mind and libidinal body, as well as the related serious blockages in the unfolding of her psychosexuality. At the same time, it served as a fertile ground for the somatization. The work that followed allowed for the creation of meaning and facilitated the reintegration of the somatic event into the chains of associations, opening the route for psychic elaboration. With time, the deepening of our understanding and further elaboration of the early trauma became possible. Towards the end of the analysis we saw the first signs of some restoration of Liona's psychosexual life through her dreams and changes she brought about in external reality.

First Discussion: Christian Seulin

While the drive concept as a theory remains widely discussed in psychoanalysis, many analysts do not use it. Some theoreticians think that what is the biological background of the psychic functioning must be considered outside psychoanalysis. In France, Jean Laplanche uses the concept of drive but only at a psychic level, focusing on the drive's source as the object to be explored with his enigmatic messages.

I am agreeing with M. Perris who, referring to Freud (1915/1957), points out that the drive is a "limit concept" between soma and psyche and has its roots in the soma. This was also Green's position.

This position does not reduce the fundamental role of the object, and many times Green wrote that object and drive were an inseparable couple.

In any case, I would like to propose some remarks and questions to Perris on a theoretical level before discussing her clinical case. In *The Interpretation of Dreams*, Freud (1900/1955) only refers to the need, and it is different to his position in the *Project of Scientific Psychology* (1895) and in the *Three Essays on the Theory of Sexuality* (1905) where one can see a differentiation between need and desire. Agreeing with many authors, I think we have to consider the role of the object in this passage from the satisfaction of the need to the satisfaction of the desire, which is the basis of the psychic functioning and the premise of fantasies. There is a very important change in this mutation because satisfaction of the need through hallucination has no effectiveness while satisfaction of desire through hallucination is the stuff of dreams and psychic life.

In her paper, Perris writes that drive is "the psychic representation of the somatic." We can certainly agree with this proposal, but I would add that it is not only that. If drive is a "limit concept" between somatic and psychic and has to be built, thanks to the object, to have a full representative state, why don't we consider that the somatic excitation from which everything is coming is not already a rudimentary form of the drive? I think that we have to talk of drive from the soma to the psyche, from excitation to drive representation. Freud (1922) only mentions that libido is the psychic energy representative of sexual drive; it is quite different.

Perris presents us the very interesting case of Liona, a young patient with somatic illnesses, gastro-intestinal troubles (history of bleeding and pre-cancerous condition), and allergy problems (eczema). She is suffering from generalized anxiety, which can be the sign of an actual neurosis.

Liona says early in the treatment that she would like to have a session each day, a desire that may indicate difficulties with regard to separation and the capacity to represent an absent object. She is in analysis five sessions a week. One could discuss in such a clinical situation the adequacy of a rigorous analytic setting. The absence of visual control of the analyst could increase anxiety. Might the frequency of sessions contribute to worsening the anxiety, increasing the dependence on the object? It does not seem so in Perris's presentation.

Thanks to the work of the analysis, Liona was relieved of much of her anxiety and somatic symptoms. We may question the way the analyst is working with her patient, as I think that a balance exists between the choice of the setting and the way the analyst is present and interpreting.

When the question of the end of analysis emerges, we clearly observe a disconnection between the patient's body and her psychic world of representation, as well as the arrival of the transference-countertransference scene of a primary trauma related to the primary object. Again, the patient feels a generalized anxiety and the return of somatic symptoms alongside a lack of representation, of associative work, and a notable extinction of feelings. Her speech is factual, and life is colorless, as she expresses. Everything turns into anxiety. Perris qualifies this period as a somatic regression.

It is very interesting to see how this anxiety and the flow of excitation without psychic expression was transmitted to the analyst. The analyst herself suffered functional digestive problems, feeling sick, fearing to receive her patient, and experiencing significant ambivalence toward her. In my experience, it is what I (2005) have called "the transmitted excitation," corresponding to the loss of qualification of affects and representation, and activated during treatment by an unthinkable danger, the return of early trauma split from the ego. In this kind of situation, it is all the construction of the drive that is regressively turned into excitation without name or meaning that the analyst is feeling. As Perris points out, the role of the work of countertransference is at stake, possessing a major place in such conjunctures. When, using her countertransference, Perris interprets the patient's fear of her weakness (i.e., the fear that Perris would not be able to receive her), she is in my opinion acknowledging the failure of the first object, that which is of great importance in such situations. I think that this interpretation was at the origin of the psychic links that the patient was able to make the following day by phone.

Perris was aptly inspired to propose a phone session when her patient was unable to come because of her sickness. In my opinion, with somatic patients, as with very severe patients, exchanges through phone calls can be helpful during critical situations. During the call, Perris offered Liona an important interpretation: "a mass of thoughts and feelings that cannot be fathomed," "and black is for mourning." The patient cried, and after this episode, the work of representation of the primary trauma could go on.

Perris shows us through her patient's nightmare how the trauma comes back at the heart of primary narcissism with the image of the piercing in the navel of a baby girl. The trauma is the disturbance of a mother during the care with her baby. We can agree with that, but I would like to discuss a point that is not clear to me. Perris refers to Laplanche and Dejours and to the lack of translation of the adult's messages as a source of excitement unbearable for the baby. Certainly in such traumas we have to consider the drive, the object, and the problem of the "bad" encounter. Inside there is already a great amount of excitation waiting for an answer; this excitation is at the drive source. Outside there is an object, and the inadequacy of this object creates more excitation. At such a conjuncture, the drive inside and the object outside are traumatic. This can explain why similar external traumas do not necessarily possess the same effect; they may be contingent upon the force of the drive push inside.

Second Discussion: Jacques Press

Hearing Perris feels to me like hearing deeply integrated French psychoanalytical thinking embedded in an English-speaking thinker, and this is a remarkable experience. I will discuss three points of her theoretical presentation before coming to her patient.

Starting from Freud's quotation in *The Interpretation of Dreams* and from Freud's (1915/1957) well-known definition of the drive, Perris makes two important points: First, she rightly underlines "the origins of the psychic in the somatic." The second point is that Freud's reference to "the original satisfaction" implies the presence of what Perris calls a "mediating object," and this object plays a major role in the establishment of the psychosomatic unity of the child and in transforming the somatic excitation into a first form of psychic representative.

I would like first to add one comment on the role of this "mediating object." In my understanding, its first role is to ensure that the *needs* of the infant are met so that a hallucinatory satisfaction of a *wish* can eventually occur. This has an important bearing on our practice when we are approaching these zones of functioning in the course of our treatments. According to

Winnicott (1954/1975), "with the regressed patient, the word wish is incorrect; instead we use the word *need*. If the patient *needs* quiet, then without it nothing can be done at all" (p. 288). Obviously, the problem is that in an adult patient, *wish* and *need* are often narrowly enmeshed with each other and that meeting a need can also satisfy a wish. But in any case, it is impossible for the analyst to continue to sit quietly in his/her chair without asking him/herself where the analytical pair is standing at this precise moment.

My second remark is linked with the preceding. In 1938, in one of his posthumous notices, Freud writes: "I am the breast. Only later: I have it, that is – I am not it" (p. 299). I will add that, between "being" and "having" the breast, there is a very painful, tricky, and nonetheless essential step: losing it. Correspondingly, according to Freud, finding the object is always re-finding it. To this, Winnicott adds that in order to be re-found the object must be destroyed in fantasy and nevertheless survive the destruction by the nascent ego. It is this continuing destruction paired with the survival of the object that makes the object – and the life – *real* for the child. In the same line of thinking, hatred has for Winnicott an important positive function, i.e., making the object real. In the context of the present discussion, one should also add that it is this whole process and the survival of the object that are the first warrants of the psychosomatic coherence of the child.

My last theoretical remark is about the concept of drive. In this regard, I am less "French" than Perris. Freud was less preoccupied than his followers with completely coherent definitions. The conception of the drive as being inseparably linked with the object is that of drives and their destiny (Freud, 1915/1957). But in *Beyond the Pleasure Principle*, five years later, things appear under another light: drives (he does not write "instincts") are forces that are present along the whole evolution, from the protozoa to the human being. I am rather inclined to leave a certain amount of openness to the Freudian concepts and not to lock them into too tightly closed boxes.

Let us now come to Liona with these points in mind. Perris describes in a very vivid manner the way in which we are involved with some patients, being taken aback while we think to intervene in an empathic matter, the feeling of incompetence they oblige us to live, and the effect it has on our own thinking process and sometimes on our own psychosomatic balance (I personally remember several bouts of severe insomnia in connection with one of my patients).

I will start from the "terrible migraine" Liona gets while her daughter is running a high fever. Perris's comment about her worries concerning her daughter meets "a cutting and sharp response back," which makes it difficult to receive. And yet I wonder: what if Liona were in some way right? Let us listen to her answer: "No, I don't think so." And she immediately adds: "anyway I always felt I exist from the neck up. I am here for you to fix my head, this would be enough and I shall be grateful."

Reading this sequence, I immediately had in mind what Pierre Marty writes about migraine: he links it with a painful inhibition of thinking due to the effort to suppress erotic and aggressive feelings. I personally feel that speaking of "erotic and aggressive" feelings is too restrictive, or rather too much defined insofar as these feelings are so crude, so undefined, so "unfathomed," as Marina rightly says in a later session. Let us put it in another way: Liona had a migraine in place of a fantasy she could not express, or of a dream she was not able to dream. And because she cannot think and dream this fantasy, she has to cut her head from her body, the reverse being equally true: because she "exists only from the neck up," she cannot dream. The result of the whole process is that the excitation returns to its bodily mooring and gives rise to the migraine.

The central question for me is the following: what is this dream that could not be dreamt? My guess is that it has something to do with a "thought." I could try to formulate it with a sentence, such as "mother and daughter can only separate from each other if and when one of them dies, separation is synonymous with death" (a stake that has important transferential implications in the context of the completion of her PhD thesis).

I feel that, in this context, Perris's supportive and empathic remark (Liona was worried about her daughter) was "felt" by Liona as a failure on the side of the analyst: she was left alone with this non-assimilable material ("felt" is not the right word; I would rather say that Liona was just, in this moment, losing every landmark), all the more since "being worried about" was probably for her at this moment very close to "killing/being killed." Interestingly enough, she reacted on two levels: on a more conscious one with her sharp reaction, and more deeply (it is deeper because it affects the thinking process itself) with her usual mode of functioning, i.e., the sever-ance of the head from the body. In other words, this was a typi-cal moment of failure on the side of the analyst, these moments that are so important and are integral parts of the analytical pro-cess. Once again, the original element Perris's observation brings is the psychosomatic dimension of such moments *for both partners*: the patient – and the analyst – take the path of a "somatic regression": disaffection, actual thinking, inability to keep a representative activ-ity, and gastro-intestinal problems.

I have just said that the unthinkable thought that took center stage during this time had to do with the equation between separa-tion and death. But herein lies a problem. In French we say: "the answer is the misfortune of the question." In other words, if we are too quick to give a representative content to this "not dreamable" material, we miss the essential point. That is, how can we help Liona give a personal form to this content, bring the somatic excitation back to the psychic side? Through her work, Perris gives us a kind of answer, an answer that is the opposite of a theoretical one: it is a proof by act.

This answer is like a coin with its two sides: On one side, the analyst has to live through herself the suffering of the patient; she has to "undifferentiate" herself from her as far as she can, and this goes actually as far as taking somatic form. On the other side of the coin, the analyst has to survive, i.e., to keep a certain amount of thinking activity, or at least try to do so. It is this sec-ond aspect that allows Perris to offer Liona an interpretation on the Monday following this horrible week: "You were anxious about what impact you had on me last Friday, you feared I became undone and I would not be here for you today." But speaking was not enough, because the need (and not only the wish) that the analyst be alive and present was so urgent: it had to be enacted both in the body through the lump and the aspiration, and in the external reality through the phone session. Only then can the response of the object acquire the quality of being *real*. And only then can Perris make her decisive intervention about "a mass of thoughts and feelings that cannot be fathomed," eventually link-ing them with the blackness and the mourning. Now the stage is ready for a more "classical" analysis, with the nightmare of the baby with the piercing, which in my opinion has a very positive value: it could be the kind of dream she could not dream when she

215

had a migraine attack. Moreover, it has to "deliver its message," a message that I feel is also that of Perris's whole paper: the early mother/infant relationship plays a central role in constructing (or distorting) the psychosomatic unity of the child.

Our Book

Experiencing the Body: A Psychoanalytic Dialogue on Psychosomatics is both the product and the reflection of how our group functions. It opens with two clinical cases. The exploration of this material served as the springboard for the theoretical thinking developed in the subsequent chapters. Another feature of our text is the presence of the commentator as a third voice in every chapter. His function is akin to that of the silent observer in the clinical workshop. It enters the scene at the end of every chapter offering a third position by commenting on the views of the two separate authors of each chapter. We chose to explore themes that appeared to us central to our topic: depression; trauma and its effects; psychosomatic investigation and treatment; drive and affects; the concepts of ideal ego, ego ideal, and superego; as well as defense mechanisms and levels of integration. The book also includes a comparative study of borderline phenomena versus somatization.

Creating the book gave us the chance to articulate the findings/contentions that arose as our work progressed, always underpinned by our sustained effort to attend to the interdependence of theory and clinical practice. Writing and discussing the book within the heterogeneity of our group brought us closer to one another's thinking and understanding of clinical work. Through effortful exploration of different and, at times, antithetical views, we arrived at rich and open exchanges and were able to articulate our propositions and findings in the field of psychosomatics. These are debated throughout our publication.

Bérengère de Senarclens

The rich exchanges mentioned earlier took us to novel vantage points and to new hypotheses. We would like to underline some of them in what follows. Our hope is that our research will generate new lines of investigation and raise questions that may be further explored in the future.

For our group, object relations theory and drive theory are fully complementary, not dissociable, and we see a constant interplay between narcissistic issues and erotic ones. In other words, we need to consider narcissistic vulnerability and its link to libidinal impulse.

What came in the foreground of our preoccupations was the "object." What do we call an object? We had to clarify our conceptions. Winnicott and Klein did not develop the same perspective in this respect. Clearly, these different views had impacted our practice. Can we conceive of a depression without an object, or in exploring depression, do we always have to consider the object? We wondered how to define a "persecutory object." Is it a traumatizing one, a chaotic one? An unfaithful, disappointing, or absent one? It seemed to us that it is related to an object that failed to be constructed internally as a constant and trustworthy one.

We considered the delicate process of the construction of the object, as well as that of the ego, insisting on the fact that such constructions are parallel processes that imply the separation of the subject and the object and the ego and the nonego, that is to say, the construction of the object in its alterity. They also imply a long "voyage" much linked to the "vicissitudes" of the mother-child relationship.

Another critical question was raised: could we envisage a specific type of depression concerning physically ill patients? What became clear was the potential link between the development of physical symptoms and the quality of the relationship to the primary objects. It appeared that a healthy "folie à deux" in very early months was an important milestone for an adequate separation process to be generated in later years. Roussillon (2016) expresses something similar, and goes further when he stresses that it is the failure of this first "choreography" between mother and infant that may generate narcissistic flaws, from which could emerge a psychosomatic pathology.

But why do we create somatic symptoms instead of psychic ones, or, more specifically, what is the nature of early traumatic relationships that might lead to somatic symptoms instead of psychic disturbances? Fotis Bobos (2019) raises the question of a qualitative specificity of somatic symptoms in relation to early traumas. It could be considered in the light of a dynamic of flight as protecting the subject against a psychic "breakdown."

This led us to the hypothesis that a "failure" in the rather primitive *oral* development might foster some somatic fragility, meaning that somatic problems would be related to an excess of excitement, dating back to very early times, to something that could not be elaborated harmoniously, nor be transformed into representation, and which, finally, remained fixed in the soma. Exploring this brought us to new developments.

It appeared to us that psychic material that could not be symbolized would pave the way for somatization *or* for acting-out, depending on the zone where the fragility originates. It seems that borderline patients, not presenting any physical symptoms, might have lived through specific difficulties dating back to a later developmental period, pertaining mainly to anal issues. Rather well adapted to life, these subjects seem to keep a sensitive wound or an early split, which under stressful and emotional circumstances might forcefully "wake up."

Along that line, we wondered how all this played out with psychotic patients. If both borderline and psychotic patients seem touched by early traumatic situations, their defenses are of a different nature. Splitting in the case of borderline states versus fragmentation in case of psychosis. This difference seems linked with the quality of the subject's ego, its strength or fragility at the time of trauma. Seulin stressed a strong relationship between melancholy and difficulties in very early development.

We all consider trauma as an essential issue when talking of physically ill patients; we view it not so much as a manifest traumatic event, but more as a subjective trauma, as it is felt by the patient. We focused on the trauma's double dimension – sexual and narcissistic, and we also arrived at the idea that what did not take place when it should have taken place constitutes a trauma in its own right.

Trauma breaks the limit between inside and outside, between subject and object. It is related to experiences which are "too much" for the subject, affecting its psychic functioning. It is related to the immaturity of the patient's ego at the time it happens. An overload of excitement makes things impossible to symbolize; therefore they remain uncontainable. As we observed, the subject's defense is often a primary splitting which might then feed the repetition mechanism; it looks as if the patient was actively repeating a failure of "attunement" of his past in a desperate attempt to try and master it. Concerning the clinical cases discussed in the group, we could adopt the idea of Ferro (2019) that if something is split off, denied or unknown, it might be somatically expressed.

Another question that attracted our attention concerned the meaning of a physical symptom. Does it have any? This idea remains controversial. We shared the view that the somatic symptom is not always "stupid." Clearly, a symptom might be "pointing" to something. Even if its meaning is not clear or easily "translatable" right away, it might somehow tell a "story" that we need to listen to, contain, and sometimes develop through a construction.

We focused at length on technical issues; certainly, our working together influenced our thoughts in that respect. We shared the sentiments of Press (2019) who posits that we should avoid thinking that something is missing in the patient but rather wonder what it is, on the analyst's side, that prevents him to understand and help the patient. This led us to place a strong emphasis on the notion of countertransference, on the need of its solid working through, that which might open a path towards approaching the traumatic zones of our patients. In other words, we should "listen" to what the patient expresses through his body or acting-out and, at the same time, listen to our own acting-out, perceptions, emotions, and bodily sensations. Bodily countertransference became central to our way of conceiving analytic work. When confronted with poor material, it is often the only way to grasp the patient's underlying emotions.

We also observed how a negative countertransference could be the expression of a patient's hidden negative transference. Often unaware of what is at stake inside of him, unaware of his aggressive move, it is through the "mirror" of the analyst's countertransference that the patient can become conscious of such emotions. We shared how hard it can be to go on thinking while enduring such feelings while, at the same time, trying to grasp them and give back to the patient something that he possibly can appropriate for himself.

Sharing clinical material led us to stress the necessity to "look for" the negative transference of the patient in its many and various forms. If not addressed and worked through, it becomes toxic, particularly with physically ill patients.

We worked on the delicate task of finding a suitable form to express these emerging emotions to the patient, of finding an adequate way to interpret the two sides of his love and hate conflict and to illustrate the two logics which are often at work in his mind:

219

a primary logic linked with his early magical thoughts – his ideal objects, and a more secondary one linked with secondary processes. Thinking of such interventions, we privileged an open and hypothetical form as opposed to an assertive one.

Some somatic patients are invested in their analysts quite massively, although, as it was the case with our patients, the analyst can feel transparent, not viewed by them as a real living person. Paradoxically, the cure on the couch can be problematic because of the strong need of these patients to somehow catch hold of their analyst perceptively. Is it their only way to fully feel his existence and possibly later develop a permanent and living internal object?

Along our journey together, we came to recognize that the emerging ability of the patient to symbolize and represent early traumatic traces, which had been automatically evacuated and split, diminished his tendency to act as well as to develop somatic symptoms. This allowed for a larger inner subjective psychic space and for a more appropriate introjection of a *third party*. Hopefully, this new capacity could help the patient to develop a better immunity. . . .

Epilogue: Marina Perris

Concluding our reflections on our work over the years, we would like to draw attention to a final critical matter, that of the distinct presence of the physical body, the soma, in the psychoanalytic work with patients who fall physically ill. Experiencing the body in psychoanalytic practice, was at the center of our explorations. At the same time, as we discussed in the Warsaw panel, the soma and its specific manifestations in analysis have also been broached in our work. The distinction between body and soma as it manifests itself in analysis is already significantly present in the analytic literature (Parat, 1995; Aisenstein, 2005, 2006; Green, 2010; Miller, 2014).

In Green's (2010) words, "The body is the libidinal body, in the broad sense (erotic, aggressive and narcissistic libido), whereas the soma refers to what is known as the biological organization" (p. 37). To our mind, the nature, extent, and possible value of this distinction in its theoretical and clinical implications invites further consideration.

Indeed, we are further suggesting that in our analytic work, we at times witness the different "presence" of the body and the soma. The differential presence gets registered *par excellence* in the transference, but even more powerfully in the analyst's countertransference. This observation seems to advocate further engagement and a promising line of investigation that can deepen our study in the field of psychosomatics.

Notes

1 Jacques Press, Fotis Bobos, Joerg Frommer, Marina Perris-Myttas, Eva Schmid-Gloor, Bérengère de Senarclens, Christian Seulin, Luigi Solano, Nick Temple.
2 The title of the paper presented in this panel was "From the Psychic to the Somatic: A Look at the Reverse Flow."

Bibliography

Aisenstein, M. (2006). The indissociable unity of psyche and soma: A view from the Paris school. *International Journal of Psychoanalysis, 87,* 667–680.

Aisenstein, M. (2013). Drive, representation, and the demands of representation. In H. B. Levine, G. S. Reed, & D. Scarfone (Eds.), *Unrepresented states and the construction of meaning: Clinical and theoretical contributions* (pp. 175–189). Karnac.

Bion, W. R. (1961). *Experiences in groups and other papers.* Routledge.

Dejours, C. (2010). Body and sexuality. *Bulletin of the European Psychoanalytical Federation, 64,* 192–203.

Ferenczi, S. (1938). Thalassa, a theory of genitality. *Psychoanalytic Quarterly,* 2 (3–4), 361–363. (Original work published 1924).

Ferro, A. (2019). *Les viscères de l'âme. Alphabet émotionnel de narrativité [The viscera of the soul: Alphabet of the emotions and narrativity].* Ithaque.

Freud, S. (1955). The Interpretation of Dreams. In J. Strachey (Ed. & Trans.), *The standard edition of the complete psychological works of Sigmund Freud* (Vol. 2). Hogarth Press. (Original work published 1900).

Freud, S. (1957). Instincts and their vicissitudes. In J. Strachey (Ed. & Trans.), *The standard edition of the complete psychological works of Sigmund Freud* (Vol. 14, pp. 117–140). Hogarth Press. (Original work published 1915).

Freud, S. (1985). "Psychanalyse" et "Théorie de la libido" [Psychoanalysis and drive theory]. In J. Altounian, et al. (Ed. & Trans.) *Œuvres complètes* (t. 16, pp. 181–208) Presses Universitaires de France. (Original work published in 1923).

Green, A. (2002). *Psychoanalysis: A paradigm for clinical thinking.* Free Association Books.

Green, A. (2010). Thoughts on the Paris school of psychosomatics. In M. Aisenstein, & E. Rappoport de Aisemberg (Eds.), *Psychosomatics today: A psychoanalytic perspective* (pp. 1–46). Karnac.

Laplanche, J. (1997). The theory of seduction and the problem of the other. *International Journal of Psychoanalysis, 78*, 653–666.

Marty, P. (1958). The allergic object relationship. *International Journal of Psychoanalysis, 39*, 98–103.

Miller, P. (2014). *Driving soma: A transformational process in the analytic encounter.* Karnac.

Miller, P. (2018). With a splinter of life. *European Psychoanalytical Federation Bulletin, 72*, 85–97.

Perris-Myttas, M. (2015). Le concept de pulsion dans le travail avec des patients somatisants [The concept of drive in the work with somatising patients]. *RFPsychosomatique, 48*, 61–75.

Press, J. (2019). *Expériences de l'informe [Experiences with the shapeless].* [Manuscript submitted for publication].

Roussillon, R. (2012). La séparation et la dialectique présence-absence [The separation and the absence-presence dialectic]. In C. Chabert (Ed.), *Les Séparations* (pp. 213–230). ERES.

Roussillon, R. (2016). Le court-circuit de la symbolisation primaire et l'incorporation mélancolique [The short circuit of the primary symbolisation and the melancolic incorporation]. In J. Press (Ed.), *Corps parlant, corps parlé, corps muet.* In Press.

Senarclens, B. de. (2016). Les métamorphoses de la "folie privée" enjeux cliniques [The metamorphosis of the "private madness," clinical stakes]. *Revue belge de psychanalyse, 68*, 59–73.

Seulin, C. (2005). L'excitation transmise [The transmitted excitement]. *Revue française de Psychanalyse, 69* (9), 203–215.

Shields, W. (2016). Affect, reverie, mourning and Bion's theory of groups in our time. In H. B. Levine, & G. Civitarese (Eds.), *The W. R. Bion tradition* (389–407). Karnac.

Smadja, C. (2005). *The psychosomatic paradox.* Free Association.

Winnicott, D. W. (1975a). Meta psychological and clinical aspects of regression within the psycho-analytical set-up. In D. W. Winnicott (Ed.), *Through paediatrics to psychoanalysis: Collected papers* (pp. 278–294). Hogarth Press. (Original work published 1954b).

Winnicott, D. W. (1975) Mind and its relation to the psyche-soma. In D. W. Winnicott (Ed.), *Through paediatrics to psychoanalysis: Collected papers* (pp. 243–255). Karnac. (Original work published 1949).

THE THREE-LEVEL MODEL

History, Mandate, Rationale, and an
Extended Case Study Exploring Change
in a Patient in Psychoanalysis
With the Three-Level Model (3-LM)

Margaret Ann Fitzpatrick Hanly, Robert White, and Siri Erika Gullestad

Part One History and Evolution
of the Three-Level Model

The Mandate

In 2009, the President of the IPA Charles Hanly proposed, and
the IPA Board established, the Project Committee on Clinical
Observation and Testing (Hanly, 2014). The goals of the Committee
(now an IPA standing professional development committee) follow:
to *explore* how clinical observations can be used to track change and
absence of change in the patient in psychoanalysis; to *explore* how the
changes observed have been brought about by the analyst's interventions and interpretations, as they change over time; to *explore* the
mechanisms of change observed in a psychoanalysis; and to *explore*
hypotheses on theories underlying interpretations and alternative
ideas for therapeutic action.

The IPA Committee on Clinical Observation is comprised of
the Chair, two Members from each of the three regions of the
IPA, and official Consultants. The Committee was chaired by
Marina Altmann de Litvan from 2010 to 2017 and by Margaret
Ann Fitzpatrick Hanly from 2017 to present. This chapter will

DOI: 10.4324/9781032656311-10

refer to the extensive work described in three published books on the Three-Level Model: *Time for Change: Tracking Transformations in Psychoanalysis – The Three-Level Model*, edited by Altmann de Litvan (Routledge, 2014) and also published in Spanish; and *Change Through Time in Psychoanalysis: Transformations and Interventions, The Three-Level Model*, edited by Fitzpatrick Hanly, Altmann de Litvan, and Ricardo Bernardi (Routledge, 2021).

The History and Evolution of the Model

The "Three-Level Model for Tracking Change in Psychoanalysis" was created by Ricardo Bernardi in 2011 (Bernardi, 2014, 2017). Committee members include experienced psychoanalysts/researchers, moderators in the Comparative Clinical Methods and End of Training Evaluation Working Parties, experts in Faimberg's Listening to the Listening Working Party, and child analysts who teach infant observation.

The early committee discussions involved wide-ranging considerations of how to observe change in the patient in psychoanalysis and how this has been done in single case studies in the literature, in supervision, and in qualitative research. What propositions about change based on what kinds of data could be made by practicing psychoanalysts who were not researchers? Two points have remained central to the model, and their significance has been further confirmed: 1) *verbatim sessions from the first week* of the analysis are important to have whenever possible; 2) there must be *sufficient intervals of time* between the next two points in the analysis from which sessions are selected to observe change and absence of change in a psychoanalysis. Bernardi articulates the thinking behind the model (Bernardi, 2014).

Two other basic ideas on method were consolidated: 1) the model would be formatted to be moderated in small group discussion in two-day meetings in IPA Societies and Regional and International Pre-Congresses; 2) the members of the group would be asked to refer to the *line-numbered text of the brief history and verbatim sessions whenever making a point*. The 3-LM group method is indebted to a Working Party method (Faimberg, 1996; Tuckett, 2008).

The core ideas of the model were tried out in practice in Montevideo (see Altmann de Litvan, 2014, pp. 35–93): 1) a *"bottom up"* exploration was carried out in the use of *three consecutive approaches or levels*, with which to have the group approach the material, *moving from the phenomenology of the session verbatim as data to conceptualization (grounded by session data), and then, to observation of what the interpretations focused on in the verbatim material and to conceptualization of mechanisms of change (grounded by session data)*; 2) the use of a reporter would summarize the group's observations on the patient's presenting problems and changes in them after two breaks in discussion, with the group adding to and correcting the verbal reports, with the goal *of correcting for each other's blind spots in the group process* (White, 2014).

Do these ideas not simply confirm that "presenting problems" are significant and change in psychoanalysis occurs gradually over time, two of the fundamentals in psychoanalytic literature? The answer is yes, but the fact that the presenting problems in those first analytic sessions are discussed over and over again *in the language of the patient* allows the group to get to know that patient's peculiar forms of expression and use them as *"anchor points"* (see Part Four) for observations of change over time. The use of the verbatim exchanges between analyst and patient in the sessions from the whole course of the analysis allows for the observation of the evolution of the analytic couple and of how change happened. As committee members worked together in 3-LM groups and in congress presentations, and in reviewing the clinical material to write case studies, we grew more confident in the usefulness of the anchor points. The actual words, tones, affects, enactments, which were the patient's presenting "expressions," as well as opening interpretations, and countertransferences, had even more information than we had expected.

In formulating the "second approach," Level Two, the group was to conceptualize the changes observed in the patient, referring again to session material. Bernardi turned to existing conceptualizations of "dimensions of psychic functioning and mental capacities," from the psychotherapy research to specify problems and change. Bernardi worked with the PDM-2 (2006) and the OPD 2 (2008) in order to create a set of questions suited to assess change in the patient in psychoanalysis, research questions suited to psychoanalysis, and having wide consensual acceptance in the mental health field (Bernardi, 2014). The 3-LM does not use the PDM and OPD as they are generally used – as a standardized diagnostic system for research – but rather to clarify the dimensions of change and absence of change over the course of a psychoanalysis. The Committee mandate was to create a model to explore observations on change that could help

225

communication between psychoanalysts, and also between psycho-analysts and colleagues in other mental health fields. Level Two questions help to differentiate the degrees and kinds of difficulties in a variety of dimensions of psychic functioning in a language that does not belong exclusively to any school in psychoanalysis. Each question adds a lens to observe specific areas of the patient's psychic functioning and mental capacities (see addendum). Some questions address the same areas of psychic functioning but from different angles.

During Level Three, the group explores the verbatim material in order to look at what the analyst's interpretations and interventions address in the patient's mind, to consider mechanisms of change, and to formulate hypotheses to observe if other interpretive strategies could have addressed material in the sessions.

Part Two Rationale for the 3-LM: Listening and Observing in Psychoanalysis

Three kinds of observation are aspired to in group discussions guided by the 3-LM: what the patient perceives and says about him/herself, the analyst's perception, enriched by his/her attitude of alert receptivity to the unconscious and intriguing aspects of the patient (Ungar et al., 2009), and the observation of the participants of the group, including their reactions.

> The clinical material is listened to with the "analytic third ear" (Reik, 1968, p. 18), the name for the instrument the analyst puts into play for his perception of unconscious communication, which reaches its greatest depth when the analyst can listen to his own voice in reaction to what the patient says.
> (Bernardi, 2014, p. 8)

The analyst, in the act of listening to his patient, "is registering the tone and the music of his voice, the silence, the language without words of the body, the noises coming from outside the consulting room," and also the analyst's "own thoughts, bodily sensations, anxieties" (Ungar, 2014, p. 98).

> Clinical reasoning is largely based upon the recognition of iterative patterns through a process that is difficult to trace and reproduce (Bernardi, 2014; Shedler & Westin, 2004). Questions from

the 3-LM aim at making this internal resonance explicit, using the group discussion as a triangulation procedure that puts together observations from diverse observers and theoretical perspectives.

(Bernardi, 2014, p. 9)

The assumption of the 3-LM method and its approach to clinical material is that, inevitably, the background psychoanalytic and personal theories (see Canestri) of the participating analysts will contribute to the focus of their observations, but also, that participants will show how the verbatim session material, which they select and read aloud, provides a good foundation for their observation.

Observation and Interpretation

Gullestad (2014) underlines the difference between observation and interpretation of clinical data, which has informed the thinking of the Committee. As stated by Freud (1914/1957), the foundation of psychoanalytic science is "observation alone" – observation is at the bottom of the theoretical structure (p. 77). Still, observations are never entirely without theory: theory informs the listening perspective of the therapist – it is through theory that the observations become psychoanalytical – "there are no unconceptualised clinical facts" (Schafer, 1994, p. 1024), i.e., ideas guide observation. However, the point is that conceptualizations are continually "checked" – and challenged – by new observations, leading sometimes to revising existing theoretical conceptualization. Tuckett (1994) claims that within our psychoanalytic field, our "standards of observation" and of "clarifying the distinction between observation and conceptualization . . . are extraordinarily low" (p. 865). As a consequence, the aim should be to "collectively take steps to clarify our focus of observation and reporting, our standards of evidence and clinical illustration" (p. 869; see also Gullestad & Killingmo, 2020). The "Project Committee on Clinical Observation and Testing" and the development of the Three-Level Model for Observing Patient Transformations represent an important step in realizing the aim of improving the observation, conceptualization, and communication of clinical psychoanalytic data. The superordinate aim is to demonstrate, both to the outside world and to the mental health authorities, that our method is capable of helping patients suffering from psychic pain (Leuzinger-Bohleber, 2014; Gullestad, 2014).

This epistemological position guides the 3-LM. Observations of important aspects of change in the patient (with verbatim evidence) rely on an ordinary scientific back and forth of deductive and inductive reasoning. The participants of 3-LM groups are asked to start (as we often do in supervision) "bottom–up" with the language of the session, referring to and reading lines from the verbatim text to indicate difficulties, interpretations, and change. Participants are then guided by the moderator (with Level Two questions) to try out concepts, which may "shed light on" or "act as a lens to clarify" more about the specifics or severity of the difficulties, always testing these tentative conceptualizations of change in the patient, using the verbatim session data from sessions taken from intervals over the course of the analysis.

Improving the Writing of Psychoanalytic Clinical Case Narratives: Expert Validation and Application of the Three-Level Model

Leuzinger-Bohleber (2014) has described the rationale for the "extended case report," or clinical narrative, which is written after the first 3-LM groups by committee members, consultants, and moderators, experienced with the model: "Established by Freud, the psychoanalytic extended case report continues to be one of the most important forms of communication in international psychoanalysis, albeit in more recent years such reports have rarely been published in international journals of psychoanalysis" (p. 124). Leuzinger-Bohleber points to those who have questioned the sufficiency of the extended case report for science, such as Thomä & Kächele (1985) who think that these reports should be checked by and complemented with other sources of evidence. However, she argues that "the comprehensive case report succeeds in conveying both to students and to a broad public 'what psychoanalysis is,' the goals it pursues and the types of transformations it effectuates in patients" (p. 124).

Part Three Extended Case Study of Ms. C.

This abbreviated psychoanalytic case study relies on material in two chapters in *Change Through Time in Psychoanalysis, Interpretation and Transformation, The Three-Level Model* (Altmann de Litvan et al., 2021; Fitzpatrick Hanly et al., 2021). The clinical narrative will demonstrate how transformation processes are explored through the 3-LM method. We present two anchor points that were regarded as expressing the patient's main difficulties and highlight how these difficulties changed during analysis. In Level Two, the narrative looks at conceptualizations of Ms. C.'s problems and changes in them with reference to verbatim session data. In the Level Three approach to the material, we present detailed verbatim material as the data for exploring how changes happened in the analysis. This account includes notes from the analyst's clinical material and reports of the 3-LM discussions.

Ms. C. was a 36-year-old single woman, half-Asian, half-Jewish, who worked as a Public Defender. She often dressed in either a "subtly or overtly sexualized and provocative style," and the analyst found herself feeling "a range of feelings from very protective to disgusted." The family immigrated from Europe to the United States when she was 6 and moved within the country shortly afterward. Her mother was hospitalized several times when Ms. C. was 10 as a result of medical problems (possibly following a hysterectomy). Some of her mother's Jewish family members were (probably) killed in the Holocaust. Her father and his extended family were from Asia; some still live there. Ms. C. said her parents were "distant" with her and often left her alone for weekends when she was a teenager, during which times she had wild parties involving sex and drugs. The analyst spoke vividly about having to contain her own anxiety during early years with Ms. C., given the very risky sexualized behaviours which she engaged in on weekends involving dangerous sex and drugs with strangers. Ms. C. started in once-a-week psychotherapy, moved to twice a week at the end of the first year of treatment, and to four times a week on the couch at the end of the second year. After a year of four-times-a-week analysis, Ms. C. announced she was leaving, and the analyst found herself saying that she knew she "had to accept this, but just could not." Ms. C. stayed on. In the fifth year of the analysis, she married, and a year later had a baby and went on a year's maternity leave.

Level One – Anchor Points and Change Points

For this version of the clinical narrative, we select two key metaphoric descriptors to use as landmarks or anchor points (also selected by the 3-LM groups) from which to assess change in the patient's problems: Ms. C. liked to be "chill"; and she engaged in many sexualized activities which actually kept her "disconnected," as exemplified in an episode in which Ms. C. proposed a "naked lunch" with a senior married male colleague.

"Chill": In the first sessions, Ms. C. said she liked to be "chill." She felt she was "above" normal needs and feelings; she liked to think of herself as self-sufficient, "on top." In this simple colloquial expression, "chill," Ms. C. conveyed core defensive strategies, "which Bernardi relates to her 'emptiness of feeling' and which Leuzinger-Bohleber elucidates in relation to early bodily experiences with a depressed mother. The 3-LM group observed that through the years of analysis Ms. C. came to understand how she had used her body to avoid feeling psychic pain and vulnerable aspects of her female body by setting up dangerous situations and trying to stay 'chill'" (Fitzpatrick Hanly et al., 2021, p. 61). The expression, an embodied metaphor, condenses her being empty of feelings and her experience of not needing another, as well as her grandiosity, her being "above" "normal needs and feelings."

Changes observed: Two years into the analysis, Ms. C. was no longer engaging in dangerous sexual encounters, and in time she expressed much more about her bodily and mental states and was able to say, "I am scared not to feel the fear." Later in the analysis, she still spoke of "layers of non-contact" in herself.

Naked lunch: In a session (while change to twice-weekly psychotherapy was being considered), Ms. C. recounted the disturbing events of the day before. One morning at breakfast, after a "blissful" night with her boyfriend M. on Valentine's Day, Ms. C. told her boyfriend that she was thinking of having a second "naked lunch" with an older, married, male colleague. M. became extremely angry. Ms. C. was still deeply distressed in her session, as she described to her analyst that she could not understand why he got so angry, that "she'd had a 'hysterical reaction' to M. yelling at her, that she'd felt 'overwhelmed.' She had 'panicked.' She thought that she was 'too opened up,' 'something went wrong.' She could not recognize her part in provoking him as she set up a repetition and felt 'overwhelmed.'" (Fitzpatrick Hanly, 2021, p. 61).

Changes observed: In the seventh year of treatment, Ms. C. (now married with a baby 5 months old) said to her analyst (speaking of the session the day before), "It was very helpful. I just thought about it a lot. . . . When things make sense, [I have] more of a physical feeling of being in touch with a certain experience." Ms. C. spoke of her experience in observing how "awkward" her mother was with her baby and expressed a sense of lack with the analyst: "In the morning I was thinking about you and me. Do we have a physical relationship? We don't have a physical relationship – being held or touched."

The telling tale Ms. C. presents about herself in the "naked lunch" episode "condenses a relationship scene in which she showed how she lived her sexuality: "Ms. C. has a 'risky' 'polymorphous' life-style involving 'sex and drugs,' casual sex with heterosexual couples, with men, with women, with a stranger 'in the hood'" (De Leon de Bernardi in Fitzpatrick Hanly et al., 2021, p. 65). She cheated on every boyfriend before her husband. "Paradoxically, both expressions 'chill' and 'naked lunch' are 'embodied metaphors' presenting core difficulties that show the estrangement of the body and the emptiness of Ms. C.'s feelings. Both metaphors are 'anchor points' from which the group could observe the unconscious aspects of Ms. C.'s relational patterns enacted in her life" and her defensive strategies, and changes in these as the analysis progressed (De Leon de Bernardi, in Fitzpatrick Hanly et al., 2021, p. 65).

"After two years of analysis, transformations began in Ms. C., who showed discomfort with, and concern about, being 'chill'" (De Leon de Bernardi in Fitzpatrick Hanly et al., 2021, p. 65). Ms. C. was able to tell her analyst more about her experience of knowing and not knowing a sexual abuse by an older male cousin who babysat for them. "I was thinking about the word dissociation. I felt in my body that numb panic." She linked "dissociation" in the moment with a bodily sensation and an affect state "panic."

Elements in these metaphoric or allegoric expressions were elaborated by Ms. C. in later sessions, and meanings that had been unconscious or split off emerged into the light of the analysis, into new language, the setting, the relationship, the transferences, and counter-transferences.

Level Two – Conceptualization:
Dissociation and Sexualization of Separation Anxiety

In selecting conceptual Level Two questions (see addendum), the moderator and the participants focus on some of the most salient observations concerning the patient's problems and the dynamics observed in Level One discussion as they are repeated and changed through the years. Level Two conceptual questions helped to clarify Ms. C.'s use of dissociation and sexualization of separation anxiety to defend against remembering traumatic states. Observations could be made in response to the questions: *"How capable is the patient of creating relationships of intimacy and reciprocity, based on stable representations which are differentiated, between herself and others?"*; *"Are defences adequate and flexible or predominantly dysfunctional, distorting or limiting internal and external experiences?"*; and *"Is the patient able to adequately regulate her impulses, her affects, and her self-esteem? and have these aspects changed?"*

The groups had reflected on Ms. C.'s lack of sustained intimacy in relationships including with the analyst. She had fantasies of remaining "chill" while compulsively engaging in "naked lunches" and "Burning Man" festivals (annual festival with art, sex, and drugs). Ms. C. compulsively had sex with young men "in the hood," with couples, and with strangers, suggesting that the fantasies of "chill" represented traumatic childhood experiences of distance from the parental figures and especially from the mother. One 3-LM group commented, "Her core conflictual relationship seems to be with the depressive mother, the 'dead mother' (in Green's sense)." "She has to have control and omnipotence." "She needs to be self-sufficient – her mother cannot supply reassurance or meet her needs" (De Leon de Bernardi, in Fitzpatrick Hanly et al., 2021, p. 67). She used her body to feel hot while trying to remain emotionally in control, "chill," and "on top."

The analyst described Ms. C.'s presenting problem, her thoughts, interpretation, and the patient's response in the first session with her patient:

> *Initially Ms. C. presented only a vague interest in growth and referred to herself as "chill"; she liked to think of herself as self-sufficient and "above" normal needs and feelings. In her first session, **I said something about how under her "chill" exterior, I sensed that there was a lot of pain.** This seemed to touch her and she started crying. I was also left with the feeling, though, that somehow this was too quick or that it had been too easy to get in or have access to her.*

The analyst unconsciously perceived that, in repeating the metaphor of "chill," she had reached a deep layer of experience and "had empathized with the patient's severe traumatization . . . the patient's despair, panic, fear of death, and distress contained" in the bodily metaphor (Leuzinger–Bohleber, in Fitzpatrick Hanly et al., 2021, p. 69).

It took time for the despair and panic to come into the analytic process. Gradually, through the analytic treatment, Ms. C. elaborated what she meant by her mother being "distant."

> The patient was able to observe how "awkward" her mother was when she held her baby son, and how she felt strange in her own body. Such a mother could not convey enough warmth to her infant in a bodily or metaphorical sense. The interactions with such a "cold," depressed primary object created an impression of unbearable coldness that the patient sought to overcome by "seeking hot sexual experiences," ("Burning Man" festival) . . . a desperate attempt at self-preservation – a kind of self-stimulation to overcome the identifications with the cold primary object.
>
> (Leuzinger–Bohleber, in Fitzpatrick
> Hanly et al., 2021, p. 72)

In the patient's history, there was a crucial unexplained loss of the object through the mother's many hospitalizations when the patient was a 10-year-old. The 3-LM group hypothesized that this might represent a separation trauma. The sexualization of separation anxiety was also linked to some "sexual abuse by the older cousin (in late latency or puberty) and promiscuous behaviour in adolescence with frequent experiences of violence. Thus, the impression of cold increasingly takes on the character of dissociation, as it is typically described in severely traumatized patients" (Leuzinger–Bohleber, in Fitzpatrick Hanly et al., 2021, p. 72). In the seventh year of the analysis, before an upcoming break, the dissociative defences have lessened, as well as the sexualization of separation anxiety. Ms. C. can speak her worry about separation: *"I guess I felt a surge of anger . . . or sadness about you going away. . . . This feeling of absence. We won't be together."*

Level Three – Foci of the Analyst's Interventions and Mechanisms of Change in the Analysis

In working with Level Three, we refer back to the difficulties and changes observed in Level One and reviewed through the conceptual lenses of Level Two, and ask *how change occurred* in Ms. C.'s struggles with dissociation and sexualization of separation anxiety. Key questions in Level Three include the following: what did the analyst's interpretations mainly address, and how did the patient respond? And what did the analyst and analysis mean to the patient?

The analyst's brief history of the analysis, written for the third 3-LM, described the opening phase of the analysis: *"her exploits seemed risky, and this, together with her nonchalant attitude, generated a sense of worry and concern in me."* The analyst writes of the particular way Ms. C. used dissociation over several years, drifting into states of non-contact with affects and sensations using habitual phrases: *"a deeply ingrained, powerful part of herself that seemed hell bent on 'smoothing' her feelings over, getting on top of . . . and making her experiences meaningless . . . whispering into her ear, 'It's all right; there's no need to be upset.'"*

The analyst reports an important interpretation when the patient said she was leaving the analysis in the third year of treatment which touched the patient and allowed her to stay:

> *In the midst of one of these seemingly fruitless discussions two weeks before she was to end, I said that I knew she was leaving, I did know it, but for some reason I couldn't accept it. I said that I had tried to accept it, I knew I needed to accept it, but that I found that I couldn't. This touched her and she stayed.*

The analyst communicated her own surprise at this unusual intervention. The analyst was not "chill," but was spontaneous in protecting the analysis rather than "smoothing over" her feelings. Four years into the analysis, Ms. C. went through a regressive movement. She met the man she married, but when the analyst left for four weeks the next summer, she arranged to be at a work-related retreat overlapping with the analyst's vacation, and her sexualized behaviour *"was in full force . . . driven and compulsive. . . . It took her quite a while for her to get out of the numb, dissociated frenzy and to get her feet back on the ground."*

The analyst's implicit ideas on change suggest she thought about containing intense anxiety over Ms. C.'s dangerous sexualized activities; about facilitating the patient's insight into her fear of being in relationship with her; about interpreting missing affects, failures to perceive danger, and the excessive dissociation. In the 3-LM group, the participant/analysts explore whether the verbatim session material *showed* that the analyst addressed these problems and interpreted in the light of her idea of what needs to change and how to bring about change in the patient.

In the "naked lunch" episode from the first hour of the psychotherapy, Ms. C. described a lovely night with her boyfriend, "serene," "settled," "sweet," "beautiful," "perfect." Then, as we described in the anchor point, she told him she was planning a second "naked lunch" with her colleague; she describes her boyfriend's rage, that she became "panicked," "overwhelmed," "hysterical." We ask, what did the analyst address in the material in this early session?

A: *It feels like it's coming out of nowhere – like one minute it's bliss and the next minute everything is falling apart – but maybe there's more to understand.*

P: *This feeling I can't be happy for too long, but I don't really believe that. I don't know. . . .*

A: *It is interesting that you said that to him, because I think you know that this would upset him and having had lunch naked with someone would upset him.*

P: *[She says she felt upset that she hadn't been more sensitive to how sensitive he is.] It didn't feel that way at the time. I had just gotten an email from him [the naked lunch colleague] – I didn't have the sense it had this hotness to it. I don't understand why he has to get so angry.*

The analyst first affirms the patient's experience, "it's bliss" and then everything "is falling apart." The patient responds, vaguely fatalistic and self-reproaching, making a series of denials: "can't be happy for too long," "don't . . . believe that," "don't know."

A: *I'm not focused on how you **should be** towards him but more whether there is anything to understand about **what goes on with you**.*

P: *[She remembers something she and I have talked about, how she'll start talking about someone else when things feel intimate.] In some way like maybe . . . It wasn't feeling uncomfortably intimate, but I think we both felt really opened up and intimate. . . . This is **maybe a strategy** I use at times without being thoughtful about it.*

A: *Aware of it.*

P: *Yes, aware of it. . . . Yes, this feels helpful to think about it that way.*

The analyst shows a non-judgemental understanding ("what goes on with you"). The patient has a flash of awareness ("This might be a strategy"), but imagines a reproach, she was not "thoughtful about it." The analyst shifts perspective; Ms. C. was not "aware of it." She thinks: "[Without being] aware of it . . . this feels helpful." It seems that the analyst's interpretation makes it safe for Ms. C. to explore how her mind works, beginning a regular attention to dissociated ideas and states.

The analyst, then, refers to the analytic frame (the starting at two sessions a week).

A: *You have said a few times that you want to talk about what's going to happen with us [two sessions], and, both times you wanted to do that, you came in, in a crisis.*

The analyst points out that Ms. C.'s coming in "in a crisis" might have been unconsciously motivated by fears about what will happen between them. The patient didn't take up the transference interpretation directly, but she began twice-weekly analytic therapy, then three times a week, and, 20 months after the "naked lunch" session, she began at four times a week.

In this third session at four times a week, Ms. C. has been at a family party with the older male cousin babysitter. She recalls the situation of possible abuse and says she is "more sure" but still has "doubt that what happened, happened." She doesn't know if she "felt upset," or if she wished "he hadn't." She cries.

A: *Maybe you wanted to know that I'm not going to lose track of you and all your feelings as you go on; that this won't be lost, that I'll hold onto it.*

Ms. C. responds with strong feelings and shifting thoughts:

P: *[Crying] . . . just because I'm not talking about it now, it's not that I'm not thinking about it. [Pause] I mean sometimes I **don't** remember. . . . It just felt helpful to hear you say that.*

In this context of dissociated memories of sexual touching, Ms. C. fears that *the analyst* thinks *Ms. C.* can't "remember," but then, Ms. C. can acknowledge gaps in her memory: "Sometimes I don't remember," and realize that she's relieved that the analyst knows that Ms. C. fears the analyst might lose track of her and her feelings,

"It helps." The analyst focuses on Ms. C.'s belief that the analyst may not keep track of her, not protect her, as Ms. C. transfers onto the analyst, her experiences with an absent, distant mother. The analyst seems to have become a new object.

One of the scary things for Ms. C., was that she could lose contact with perceptions of danger.

A: *I think about you at this party Saturday, or when your cousin touched you, or when you left here Friday, feeling abandoned by me — like out there on your own, and feeling how can this happen and no one's looking out for you.*

P: *I did feel on Friday — we did talk about me going to my cousin's close to the end. I did feel like it was like, "OK . . . good luck."*

The analyst interprets Ms. C.'s sense that had she'd sent her away into danger without caring and the patient can respond, yes, it felt like a dismissive, "good luck." The patient is able to tolerate ambivalence, holding contradictory feeling states, safe enough to say she felt dismissed. At the end of the session, the analyst interprets the patient's anger at not being protected, *"It sounds like you feel unprotected by and angry at them [her friend and parents] and me also, and then you turn to men"* (end of session). The analyst's interpretations focused on a sequence: the patient's feeling unprotected and angry at parents and analyst, and then turning to a sexualized contact. A gradual change is observed in Ms. C.'s deepening capacity to re-experience the object relational traumata and overstimulation, brought about by the interpretations in the safety of a non-judgmental space.

During this period, Ms. C. got married and became pregnant. In the last session presented in this material, Ms. C. speaks of a thought she has when feeding her 5-month-old baby: "I haven't had any safe physical relationship that wasn't sexual"; she says her relationship with her baby "was the first one." She realizes: "I didn't have a very physical relationship with my parents. Anything physical is or could become sexual." She tells the analyst that the baby had had a

big meltdown with my mom, and it was pretty hard for her and him. I was really upset, I felt bad that she had to deal with it on her own. Like I was worried that like she wouldn't want to take care of him anymore. Like he's too much.

She had the "feeling my mom would be overwhelmed, frantic," and worried "what that would mean about her taking care of him in the future." Her mother had been unable to settle the baby who was crying frantically.

In this phase of the analysis, Ms. C. started wondering about the physical relationship with the analyst. The analyst asks, *"Around something in particular?"* And the patient tells her:

> when I'm reading – by myself – it's a very familiar feeling of reading – this would be common in any book – when the character is yearning. In this vampire book that I'm reading, the guy is yearning for blood but it seems sexual.

The analyst asked if the vampire is *"yearning for blood or a person? Is he yearning for a person?"* Ms. C. first stays with the physical/sexual "a focus and warmth in the genital region and a pressure that wants to be relieved . . . longing and yearning."

Ms. C. then says she feels safer reading and feeling these things than "actually doing something sexual." She's quiet for a while and then says with a different focus,

> the clock's positioned towards someone else. Why didn't you move it back? . . . Before that I had a flash of something sexual with you, still in the white tank top. It's right here and I'm pulling you towards me – our mouths. It also felt scary, and unsafe.

The analyst makes an interpretation, which is central to a main focus of her attention:

A. *Maybe what we're seeing is you start to have a feeling in your body, maybe a yearning, a feeling of loss, anger, like when you felt like the clock was turned towards someone else and you imagined me with someone else, and then this fantasy happens, a sexual fantasy, or a sexualized fantasy, that kind of obliterates that, your feelings, that is.* (Ms. C. is crying.)

This kind of here-and-now transference interpretation appears to have had a deep effect on the patient's psychic functioning, on her relationships (inside and outside the analysis) and on her sexuality, over time. The patient did not take up the transference directly but used the transference to feel contained and held. The patient began to gain more insight into disavowed affects and more access to fantasy, as we see in later sessions.

Eight years into the analysis, the analyst was going to leave for a week, in a week. The patient says she slept "horribly" and when she woke, she "*felt like there was an earthquake. I was sure my bed was vibrating.*" She was "*a little panicked, that heartbeat feeling – but feeling doubt too.*" She wonders if she had imagined an earthquake. She thought about the upcoming break because she was desperately trying to keep a feeling of "*stability before the break.*" She hoped she would not be "*feeling abandoned by you when you were gone,*" but "*now it seems like the whole sense of that seems shaky, like the bed. Like scared . . . I can't trust, I can't rely on you.*" This is a key development in her ability to speak about the negative transference, related to the core object relational traumata (the immigrant parents, the depressed mother, hospitalized, and a remote father, leaving her alone to wild parties in adolescence). And we see a greater capacity for symbolization, for metaphor: Ms. C. feels "*abandoned . . . shaky like the bed . . . scared.*"

The analyst asks, "Do you know what [your feelings] are?" After a long pause, when the analyst does not speak, Ms. C. brings new thoughts.

P: *When I was awake, I was thinking about you. I wonder what time she goes to bed? I don't imagine you go to bed at 9:00. I have an image of people who go to bed at 9. I wonder, what time do they eat dinner? How much time do you see your kids and how annoyed do you get if you spend a lot of time with them?* [She's quiet.]

The patient showed a curiosity about the analyst and her kids, suggesting she could now see the analyst as a separate person with her own concerns and motivations. After a few clarifications, the analyst made a long transference interpretation:

A: *Maybe in the middle of the night there was initially some sense of feeling and alone and then thinking of me and not knowing what I am doing or where I am, and then maybe that was connected with knowing I am going to be away and . . . some sense of separation and incompleteness. Some area where we are not overlapping. Then that's hard to fathom and that's scary and vulnerable and, then, it becomes more about . . . to not have that feeling.*

239

The analyst pays attention to Ms. C.'s feeling "alone," her fear of separation, a new sense that they do not "overlap" entirely, (ego-object differentiation), and her wish not to have the feeling (to disavow affect again), all placed in the transference. The patient response is to become aware of new feeling states:

P: *I guess I felt a surge of anger . . . or sadness about you going away, I guess.*
A: *Yeah, what did you feel?*
P: *A flash of, oh I could just cry. It was very fleeting. I guess feeling tenderly towards myself for having a hard time having feelings. . . .*
P: *This feeling of absence. We won't be together.*

A 3-LM group noted that the analyst did not interpret that Ms. C. might have felt excluded by the idea of the analyst and her husband, as an Oedipal couple, going to bed at 9 or 10. The analyst and Ms. C. were able to talk about the years of dangerous sexual experiences and how dissociated she was during them and how scary many of them were. Ms. C. was able to see and think about how dissociated her mother was and how that has affected her.

Part Four Three-Level Model: Description

The 3-LM is a flexible model. Its aim is to ask more and more useful, cogent, and accurate questions that help to understand the changes in patients in analysis (see Fitzpatrick Hanly et al., 2021).

Level One and Group Process

In Level One discussion, the group participants are asked to listen to the material read by the analyst and to describe in plain language observations of the patient's difficulties and change and no change in the patient guided by the following 3-LM questions (Bernardi, 2014): "*a) How does the patient use the analyst? b) How does the patient use the analyst's interventions? c) How does the patient use his/her own mind and body during the session?*," and can changes be observed? Another set of questions is related to exploring changes in the life of the patient, a controversial focus for psychoanalysts. "*Is it possible to observe changes in the patient's capacity to love and sexuality; family and social relationships; occupation and leisure; interests and creativity; symptoms and subjective well-being?"* And another question asks, *"Which parts of the clinical material had a special resonance for the participants of the group and can be considered as anchor points that make it possible to track changes in the patient?"*

During the hours of reading the words of the patient and the analyst, the participants strive to get a sense of this particular patient in this analysis speaking in ordinary language. Thus, Level One is referred to as a "phenomenological approach" to the material. Shared resonances in the group open new paths of inquiry, achieving a certain state of daydreaming or "transformation in dreaming" (Ferro, 2009). The analytic experience is often grasped through the inner resonance of participants with the clinical material, and the experience may be expressed through metaphors created in the analytic field (de León de Bernardi, 2013), a quasi-artistic process (Altmann, 2008; Birksted-Breen, 2012). The group is asked to examine the clinical material independently of the analyst's point of view, and as much as possible, independently from conceptual language and theories. Participants pay attention to how the clinical material affects them, and to how a dynamic may be playing out in the group process. Often a phenomenon in the group process is brought into the discussion for reflection by the moderator, reporter, or other member of the group.

Observations and intuitions must be grounded in the verbatim of the session material, with lines of the clinical text read for validation. Over the years of moderating 3-LM groups, the committee and consultants have been struck by the way a group of analysts from different countries and cultures does see so much in common. "Group think" is considered as possibly leading to bias. However, when material from the analysis of Ms. C. was presented to three groups, participating analysts focused on the same anchor points (the naked lunch, the wish to be chill) and observed the changes in the core presenting problems. In "A Dialogue between 3-LM Moderators and Presenters," the analyst presenter of the case of Ms. C. writes:

[R]equiring participants to provide evidence (a line number) for any statement that they make about the case provides a structure that ensures rigor. It creates a tight working experience of people thinking together about a case without anyone being able to privilege and impose their own theory on the material. This also ensures a level playing field among the group members; no matter how brilliant anyone's formulation, it has to be grounded in the text.

(Fitzpatrick Hanly & Altmann de Litvan, 2021, p. 238)

Selection of Anchor Points and Group Process

In the course of the Level One discussion, through referring to the verbatim sessions, key presenting problems *in the language of the patient* are gradually honed in upon. The "anchor point" expressions are vivid, unique to a specific analytic patient (dynamics, states of mind, self-images), and repeated at later points the analysis, a repetition which permits the observation of change in specific dimensions of psychic functioning (e.g., the metaphor for self as "chill" and the "naked lunch" story).

The moderator and reporter may notice possible anchor points when reading the sessions before the 3-LM group meets. However, good anchor points for observing change are always discovered by the group of psychoanalytic minds, resonating to "telling" expressions in the analytic material, when passages are paused over, puzzled over, returned to, in the discussion. The anchor points, which the reporter writes up in the break and presents for revision, are further *validated (or not)* by the group as the two-day discussion proceeds. Later readings of the material and discussion by committee members preparing a clinical narrative may bring out a new anchor point related to a key change point in the patient and analysis when an early expression is more clearly understood. The model is open to the selection of other anchor points which allow the observation of change in psychoanalysis, based on session data.

An anchor point may be a key metaphor, an enactment, a gesture, or a story (which has allegorical meaning) told in the first sessions that captures core conflicts, defensive strategies, hints of trauma, or deficits in psychic structure which are elaborated, shifting over the years of the analysis. Another way to put it is that good anchor points offer highly condensed depictions of the patient's core dynamics on entering the analysis. In the extended case study of Ms. C., three 3-LM groups selected the same anchor points and observed several of the same change points. However, consensus is not essential and there may be significant differences about what to prioritize as the patient's central problem or what passages best show change or absence of change in functioning. What is essential is that sufficient relevant data from three separate phases of the analysis can ground well-defined clinical thinking on difficulties and change. Responses to the material and observations on change made by one participant, or several, can correct for another participant's blind spot. As the group discusses these differences, a more complex idea of the patient and the analysis emerges. 3-LM groups often become quite passionate as they become immersed in the material.

We emphasize that group discussion at Level One uses only the language of the session and ordinary language in a bottom-up approach, so that phenomena that do not easily fit into a theory are kept in play (Bernardi, 2017). The reading and re-reading of the words of patient and analyst (first read by the analyst in the room) touches the preconscious of the participants.

The Committee has noted that the analyst may have (consciously or unconsciously) considered telling indicators of change through the years of the analysis, patterns repeated, that influenced the analyst's interpretation and selection of sessions. In this light, questions about possible "bias" in this observational research are under discussion by the committee: is the selection of anchor points by the 3-LM groups influenced by the moderator? Is the emergence of anchor points the result of conscious or pre-conscious ideas on patterns of change in the analysis by the analyst?

Level Two: Conceptualization of
Difficulties and Observed Change or Absence of Change

In Level Two discussion, questions are raised to help conceptualize the main dimensions of the difficulties in which change or absence of change has been observed. These questions are rooted in psychodynamic categories based on systems proposed by the Psychodynamic Diagnostic Manual (PDM, 2006) and the Operationalized Psychodynamic Diagnosis (OPD, 2008). The moderator and reporter meet in the break to look over the summary report on the anchor points and change points to see which conceptual questions are most relevant to begin with. This may also create a bias; however, the participants are also reading the questions and may select other conceptualizations to consider over several hours.

Level Two can highlight the unevenness of transformations, change in certain areas of functioning, as well as no change or deepening of the conflict in the patient's life, the associations, or the transference. The questions in Level Two of the 3-LM selected and re-formulated by Bernardi from the PDM-2 (2006) and the OPD-2 (2008) focus not on symptoms or signs of well-being, but on the core concepts of psychoanalytic theory which underlie them. Even these conceptually oriented questions are "expressed in the most theoretically unsaturated way possible," in ways that sharpen observations of the verbatim session material, so "analysts from different analytic traditions can then reframe ideas in the light of their own theoretical preferences" (Bernardi, 2014, p. 15). This makes it possible to discover that different theoretical concepts sometimes refer to the same clinical phenomenon, easing communication between analysts identifying with different theoretical traditions. The diagnostic systems from which the questions are selected

> aim at operationalizing their concepts, making them user friendly for clinicians from different traditions. The OPD-2 states that a challenge in doing this is not to lose conceptual content in order to gain consensus, and, therefore, proposes to use the "smallest common multiple" among the different meanings of the concepts.
> (Bernardi, 2014, p. 13)

The first group of questions on the "subjective experience of illness" considers the patient's experience of suffering, the degree to which a patient can acknowledge his or her problems and imagine change. (*What are the patient's subjective experiences, beliefs, and expectations about his/her problems and treatment? How much does (s)he recognize his/her problems? How much can (s)he foresee possibilities of change?*)

The second group of questions on "patterns of interpersonal relationships" has its origin both in the classical notion of transference and countertransference and refers to changes in relational patterns outside the analysis. (*How are the interpersonal relationships of the patient, especially in the bonds which imply closeness and intimacy? How does the patient experience others, and how does she experience herself in relation to others – both in transference-countertransference and in the other meaningful bonds?*) Tracking change from the "Naked Lunch" episode, when Ms. C. seemed to have no clue about how she provoked her boyfriend, was clarified through discussion of these conceptual questions.

The third group of questions explores the patient's "main intrapsychic conflicts." Change can be seen when the patient is capable of a more flexible use of defences and less use of defences that distort or restrict internal or external experience. (*What are the main conflicts, e.g., individuation vs. dependency; submission vs. control; need for care vs. self-sufficiency; conflict in self-worth, in guilt; Oedipal conflict; identity conflict? Which are the dominant unconscious fantasies that can be inferred from conflicts and relational patterns? Are the prevailing defences flexible or dysfunctional, distorting or limiting internal and external experiences?*) Several conflicts were considered, but what emerged as a core issue was that (having suffered through childhood object relational trauma) Ms. C. used a dissociative defence in a dysfunctional and distorting way, and that change occurred as she could own affects and impulses and dissociate less.

The fourth group of questions, those on the patient's "mental and personality functioning," explores vulnerabilities, fragilities, deficits, and/or developmental arrests in the patient. The four dimensions, or categories, follow the OPD-2 (2008) criteria.

The first dimension refers to the patient's capacity to perceive what occurs in his own mind and to build, based on that, an integrated and differentiated sense of personal identity. (*How capable is the patient of adequately perceiving her own internal states and those of others? Is she able to empathize, tolerating and understanding the existence of different points of view? Does she have an integrated feeling of her own identity, open to the possibility of unconscious aspects? What are the characteristics of the identifications – especially pathological ones?*) These questions acted as a lens to clarify Ms. C.'s desperate struggle to connect, while not in contact with her own feeling states, and not seeing others' points of view. Her identification with a depressed "distant" mother from a traumatic background could be observed as Ms. C. separated from her mother.

The second dimension refers to the capacity to regulate impulses, affects, and self-esteem, as well as to establish an adequate emotional balance between the needs of the self and the needs of others. Ms. C.'s compulsive sexual activities and paucity of affect were focussed on through this lens.

The third dimension asks: *How rich is the dialogue with herself and others, based on affective experiences, bodily self, fantasies, dreams, sexuality, symbolic representations, and capacity to play and creativity?*

245

The fourth structural dimension asks: *How deep and stable and differentiated are the relationships with internal and external objects? How well can she begin and end relationships and tolerate separations? How does (s)he handle relationships which imply the existence of a third?* These capacities contribute to self-identity and self-direction, as well as to empathy and intimacy. We saw that Ms. C. compulsively engaged in dangerous sexual acts when threatened with separation, and that changes occurred as transference interpretations addressed buried feelings of being "lost track of" and dismissed at times of separation from the analyst.

The fifth group of questions asks if there is an identifiable disturbance that has affected the analysis, and asks about the level of personality organization: *"How severe are the disturbances of personality functioning? How much is analytic work conditioned by the structural vulnerabilities of mental functioning?"* (Bernardi, 2014, pp. 16–18).

Level Three: Therapeutic Foci and Mechanisms of Change

In Level Three, the questions for discussion ask what the analyst has focused on in the patient's material and whether there is a change in what the analyst focused on in her interpretations over the course of the analysis.

1. *What did the analyst's interventions address in the material? Did the foci of interventions change over the course of the analysis? What can be observed about the impact on the patient of the different foci of interventions, in different phases in the analysis? What moments and interventions were especially moving for the patient? And why?*
2. *What are the possible change mechanisms/curative factors in this analysis, e.g., insight, corrective emotional experience, analyst as a "new object"/ new model, affirmation, containment, reconstruction? (The analyst's intentions may be different from what we, as outside observers, see as factors in the change observed.)*
3. *What parts of the clinical material were not addressed by the analyst? And what other foci of interventions could the 3-LM group hypothesize might have been useful?*

The Committee revised the Level Three questions slightly to add a question on interventions that were especially moving for the patient, to distinguish mechanisms of change from therapeutic action, and to observe more specifically if some aspect of the clinical material was not focussed on by the analyst's interventions in order to formulate alternative hypotheses. The aim is to do a microanalysis of the relationship between intervention and change, contributing to the study of mechanisms of change. The most speculative part of Level Three discussion is to hypothesize on the theories underlying patterns of interventions by the analyst, and to speculate on whether another set of interventions rooted in concepts a participant brings from another analytic theory would have addressed some unaddressed aspect of the material. Again, specific references to the verbatim material must be made in this phase of the discussion.

Current Initiatives

Members of the committee and consultants have adapted the model to new uses in developing clinical narratives based on the work of the committee groups' re-thinking observations of change and how change happens in "a third look," illustrated in the extended case studies of Ms. C., written for this chapter and in Fitzpatrick Hanly, Altmann de Litvan, and Bernardi's (2021) recent edited collection in which committee members have further articulated how the Three-Level Model can be used as a "clinical research tool."

The Three-Level Model has been adapted in IPA training programs to help candidates write reports and clinical papers for graduation. As a "Professional Development" Committee of the IPA, the central goal remains to offer 3-LM clinical observation groups at Regional Meetings and IPA Pre-Congresses, and in IPA Societies to help analysts track observations of change and no change in the psychoanalytic patient.

In exploring the transformations in psychoanalysis, the Three-Level Model shares a goal with the wider mental health field. In this age of "evidence-based psychotherapy," it is important to show that psychoanalysis can promote meaningful transformations and can describe how change occurs (Altmann de Litvan, Bernardi, & Fitzpatrick Hanly, 2021). A current focus of the committee is to explore the nature of the evidence in the verbatim sessions, to show how transformations are facilitated by interventional strategies and patterns of interventions. Committee members have proposed a tentative framework to assess the weight of evidence (low, moderate, or high) combining key dimensions of clinical materials. A chapter on method in Committee members' recent book discusses matters of evidence more broadly and from the point of view of the philosophy of science (Bernardi, Perez & Hanly, 2021).

The Three-Level Model focusses on comparing the initial points and change points in a psychoanalytic process. The Committee has a collection of clinical materials and case reports from different regions and analytic cultures and is discussing how to approach the comparative analysis of change, absence of change, and how change happens in three analytic cases. The Committee has opened discussion on the exploration of change in "specimen" cases, defined in the research literature. We are engaged in a gradual work in progress.

Bibliography

Alliance of Psychoanalytic Organizations. (2006). *Psychodynamic diagnostic manual*. Wiley.

Altmann, M. (Ed.) (2014). *Time for change: Tracking transformations in psychoanalysis: The Three-Level Model*. Karnac.

Altmann de Litvan, M. (2008, August). Cómo se da el nacimiento del paciente en la mente del analista [The emergence of the patient in the analyst's mind] [Paper presentation] Sixteenth annual conference of the Uruguayan Psychoanalytic Association, Montevideo, Uruguay.

Altmann de Litvan, M., Bernardi, R., & Fitzpatrick Hanly, M. (2021). The Three-Level Model: Is the Three-Level Model a clinical research tool? In M. Altmann de Litvan (Ed.), *Clinical research in psychoanalysis: Theoretical basis and experiences through Working Parties* (pp. 172–182). Routledge.

Altmann de Litvan, M., Fitzpatrick Hanly, M., & White, R. (2021). Underlying clinical thinking on change and therapeutic action. In M. Fitzpatrick Hanly, M. Altmann, & R. Bernardi (Eds.), *Change through time in psychoanalysis: Transformations and interpretations: The Three-Level Model* (pp. 34–59). Routledge.

Bernardi, R. (2014). The Three-Level Model (3-LM) for observing patient transformations. In M. Altmann (Ed.), *Time for change: Tracking transformations in psychoanalysis – the Three-Level Model* (pp. 3–34). Karnac.

Bernardi, R. (2017). A common ground in clinical discussion groups: intersubjective resonance and implicit operational theories. *Int. J. Psychoanal.*, *98*, 1291–1309.

Bernardi, R., Perez, L., & Hanly, C. (2021). Assessing strengths and limitations of clinical evidence in a psychoanalytic clinical material. In M. Fitzpatrick Hanly, M. Altmann, & R. Bernardi (Eds.), *Change through time in psychoanalysis: Transformations and interpretations: The Three-Level Model* (pp. 281–305) Routledge.

Birksted-Breen, D. (2012). Taking time: The tempo of psychoanalysis. *Int. J. Psycho-Anal.*, *93* (4), 819–835.

Canestri, J. (Ed.). (2006). *Psychoanalysis: From practice to theory.* John Wiley and Sons.

De León de Bernardi, B. (2013). Field theory as a metaphor and metaphors in the analytic field and process. *Psychoanal. Inq.*, *33* (3), 247–266.

De León de Bernardi, B. (2021). Key metaphors of the self as a multiple bridge for clinical research. In M. Altmann de Litvan (Ed.), *Clinical research in psychoanalysis: Theoretical basis and experiences through Working Parties* (pp. 134–148). Routledge.

Faimberg, H. (1996). Listening to listening. *Int. J. Psycho-Anal.*, *77*, 667–677.

Ferro, A. (2009). Transformations in dreaming and characters in the psychoanalytic field. *International Journal of Psychoanalysis*, *90*, 209–230.

Fitzpatrick Hanly, M. A. (2019). Transformations in female bodily experiences and bodily metaphors. *International Journal of Psychoanalysis*, *100* (5), 1031–1033.

Fitzpatrick Hanly, M. A., Altmann, M., & Bernardi, R. (Eds.) (2021). *Change through time in psychoanalysis, transformations and interventions: The Three-Level Model.* Routledge.

Fitzpatrick Hanly, M. A., Altmann de Litvan, M. (2021) A Dialogue between 3-LM Moderators and Presenters. In M. Fitzpatrick Hanly, M. Altmann, & R. Bernardi (Eds.), *Change through time in psychoanalysis, transformations and interventions: The Three-Level Model.* (pp. 234–243). Routledge.

Fitzpatrick Hanly, M. A., De Leon de Bernardi, B., & Leuzinger-Bohleber, M. (2021). Bodily metaphors as anchor points in facilitating change. In M. Fitzpatrick Hanly, M. Altmann, & R. Bernardi (Eds.), *Change through time in psychoanalysis, transformations and interventions: The Three-Level Model* (pp. 60–75). Routledge.

Freud, S. (1957). On narcissism: An introduction. In J. Strachey (Ed. & Trans.), *The standard edition of the complete psychological works of Sigmund Freud* (Vol. 14, pp. 67–102). Hogarth Press. (Original work published 1914).

Gullestad, S. E. (2014). Close to observation: Some reflections on the value of the Three-Level Model for observing patient transformation to study change. In M. Altmann (Ed.), *Time for change: Tracking transformations in psychoanalysis: The Three-Level Model* (pp. 163–184). Karnac.

Gullestad, S. E., & Killingmo, B. (2020). *The theory and practice of psychoanalytic therapy: Listening for the subtext.* Routledge.

Hanly, C. (2104). Foreword. In M. Altmann (Ed.), *Time for change: Tracking transformations in psychoanalysis – The Three-Level Model* (pp. ix – xxiv). Karnac.

Leuzinger-Bohleber, M. (2014). Depression and trauma: The psychoanalysis of a patient suffering from chronic depression. In M. Altmann (Ed.), *Time for change: Tracking transformations in psychoanalysis – The Three-Level Model* (pp. 122–162). Karnac.

OPD Task Force. (2008). *Operationalized psychodynamic diagnosis manual of diagnosis and treatment planning.* Hogrefe and Huber.

Reik, T. (1968). Theodor Reik speaks of his psychoanalytic technique. *Amer. Imago, 25* (1), 16–20.

Schafer, R. (1994). The conceptualisation of clinical facts. *Int. J. Psychoanal., 75,* 1023–1030.

Shedler, J., & Westin, D. (2004). Refining DSM-IV personality disorder diagnosis: Integrating science and practice. *American Journal of Psychiatry, 161,* 1350–1365.

Thomä, H., & Kächele, H. (1985). *Lehrbuch der psychoanalytischen Therapie [Textbook of Psychoanalytic Therapy].* Springer.

Tuckett, D. (1994). The conceptualization and communication of clinical fact in psychoanalysis. *Int. J. Psycho-Anal., 75,* 865–870.

Tuckett, D. (Ed.), Basile, R., Birksted-Breen, D., Böhm, T., Denis, P., Ferro, A., Hinz, H., Jemstedt, A., Mariotti, P., & Schubert, J. (2008). *Psychoanalysis comparable and incomparable: The evolution of a method to describe and compare psychoanalytic approaches.* Routledge.

Ungar, V. (2014). Tracking patient transformations: The function of observation in psychoanalysis. In M. Altmann (Ed.), *Time for change: Tracking transformations in psychoanalysis: The Three-Level Model* (pp. 97–121). Karnac.

Ungar, V., Koritar, E., Jacobs, T., Bolognini, S., Ungar, V., Rolland, J. & Turgeon, A. (2009). The core of the psychoanalytic practice. *Canadian Journal of Psychoanalysis, 18,* 141–146.

White, R. (2014). A report on Paula with "no history." In M. Altmann (Ed.), *Time for change: Tracking transformations in psychoanalysis: The Three-Level Model* (pp. 227–236). Karnac.

ADDENDUM LEVEL 2 QUESTIONS ADAPTED FROM OPD-2 (2008) (SEE BERNARDI, 2014)

TABLE 2. *QUESTIONS FOR LEVEL 2 Discussion: DIMENSIONS OF CHANGE*

1) *SUBJECTIVE EXPERIENCE OF ILLNESS AND CONTEXTUAL FACTORS*

1A) What are the patient's subjective experience, beliefs and expectations about his/her problems and treatment? How much does (s)he recognize his/her problems? How much does (s)he foresee possibilities of change? To what extent do patient and analyst agree regarding the expected transformations?

1B) Do contextual factors exist which affect the therapeutic process? (For example, crisis situations, traumatic experiences, somatic illnesses, drugs, etc.? How capable is the patient to face these situations?)

1C) How have these aspects changed? How much has the patient's understanding of his/her problems and therapeutic possibilities modified?

2) PATTERNS OF INTERPERSONAL RELATIONSHIP *and how have they changed?*

2A) How are the interpersonal relationships of the patient, especially in the bonds which imply closeness and intimacy?

2B) How does the patient experience others and how does he experience himself in relation to others? How do others experience the patient and how do they experience themselves in relation to the patient? (Both in transference-countertransference as in the other meaningful bonds.)

2C) To what extent can I relate the patient's current relational patterns to the experiences lived in his/her childhood and with the bonds that he establishes with the analyst?

2D) How have these aspects changed?

3) MAIN INTRAPSYCHIC CONFLICTS *and how have they changed?*

3A) What are the main conflicts (e.g., individuation vs dependency; submission vs control; need for care vs self-sufficiency; self-worth, guilt, Oedipal conflict, identity conflict)? Which are the dominant unconscious fantasies that can be inferred from conflicts and relational patterns?

3B) The prevailing defences are adequate and flexible or dysfunctional, distorting or limiting internal and external experiences?

3C) How have these aspects changed?

4) STRUCTURAL ASPECTS OF MENTAL FUNCTIONING

4A)   What is the level of mental functioning in the following areas? Are there signs of change?

4.A.1. PERCEPTION OF SELF AND OTHERS. IDENTITY.

How capable is the patient of adequately perceiving his/her own internal states and those of others?

Is (s)he able to empathize, tolerating and understanding the existence of different points of view?

Does (s)he have an integrated feeling of his/her own identity, open to the possibility of unconscious aspects?

What are the characteristics of the identifications (especially pathological ones)?

Does (s)he manage to connect with his/her past and give direction to his/her life, with a sense of agency and short and long term wishes and goals?

4.A.2. AFFECTIVE REGULATION: Is the patient able to adequately regulate his/her impulses, affects, and self-esteem? Do his/her ideals and values help him/her to handle his/her emotions? Does (s)he manage to regulate his/her need of self-esteem when facing internal and external demands? How much does (s)he achieve an adequate balance between his/her own interests and those of the others?

4.A.3. INTERNAL AND EXTERNAL COMMUNICATION. SYMBOLIZATION. How rich is the dialogue with him/herself and the others, based on affective experiences, bodily self, fantasies, dreams, sexuality, symbolic representations, and capacity to play and creativity?

4.A.4. ATTACHMENT WITH INTERNAL AND EXTERNAL OBJECTS.

How deep and stable and differentiated are the relationships with internal and external objects?

How much can (s)he start and finish relationships and tolerate separations?

How does (s)he handle relationships which imply the existence of a third one?

4.B) How have these aspects changed?

5) **TYPE OF DISORDER**

5.A) Is it possible to identify a type of personality disorder or other kind of mental or bodily disorder?

5.B) How severe are the disturbances of personality functioning? How much is analytic work conditioned by the structural vulnerabilities of mental functioning?

5.C) How have these aspects changed?

IN ITS MORE THAN 20 YEARS OF EXISTENCE, WHAT CONTRIBUTIONS HAVE WORKING PARTIES BROUGHT TO PSYCHOANALYSIS AND PSYCHOANALYTIC RESEARCH?

Patrizia Giampieri-Deutsch

Specific and Nonspecific Contributions of Working Parties to Psychoanalysis

This closing chapter returns to the overall title question of the volume and provides a summary overview of the remarkable impact, both intended as well as unintended, of Working Parties on psychoanalysis and its research. On the part of Working Parties, the specific results achieved on their chosen topics display an unquestionably wide range of goal-oriented contributions, which arise from their steady ongoing activities. Additionally, a variety of beneficial general effects on the psychoanalytic community should also be taken into consideration, some of which are, on the part of Working Parties, entirely or partly unlooked for.

Plurality

In 2000, David Tuckett, the then president of the European Psychoanalytic Federation (EPF), called for a "Ten-year scientific initiative." Eight years later, his introductory chapter, "On difference,

DOI: 10.4324/9781032656311-11

discussing differences and comparison," to a book on the *Working Party on Comparative Clinical Methods* (WPCCM) (Tuckett et al., 2008) resumed Arnold Cooper's (2003) somewhat theatrical characterization of "orthodoxy" in psychoanalysis as an "intellectual reign of terror," pointing out that "[a]ll psychoanalytic groups have experienced charismatic authority, with the problem intensified by the integral role of training analysis, which have inevitable emotional and social consequences within societal life" (Tuckett, 2008a, p. 6).

Up to a point, his critique can be considered plausible. However, it needs to be put into perspective. A previous remark of Robert Michels brought up that the crucial issue of training is hardly its social psychology: "All organized educational systems struggle with conflicts over power, autonomy, and authoritarianism and the problems of psychoanalysis in this arena are not unique" (Michels, 2007, p. 987).

It is common knowledge that Freud (1921c/1955), in *Group psychology and the analysis of the Ego*, rejects the contrasting juxtaposition of

individual psychology and social or group psychology. . . . In the individual's mental life someone else is invariably involved, as a model, as an object, as a helper, as an opponent; and so from the very first individual psychology, in this extended but entirely justifiable sense of the words, is at the same time social psychology as well.

(p. 69)

Introducing psychoanalysts to this work's seminal distinction between the ego and the ego ideal and the specific processes of identification with the leader of a group putting himself or herself in the place of the ego ideal of each member of the group, would be like carrying coals to Newcastle. Therefore, I expect I am stating the obvious when I say that rather than distinctive or unique to psychoanalytic training, these specific processes of identification with a leader and their consequences are indeed highly ubiquitous and manifest themselves in workplaces, academia, politics, and sports associations, to name just a few arenas where such dynamics are seen to arise.

I will return later to the successful efforts of the Working Parties to deepen the understanding of training processes and subsequently greatly contribute to their improvements.

257

A Threat to the Unity?

While stating that the capacity of psychoanalysis to impose authority has increasingly weakened, to substantiate his own claim Tuckett adds in reference to Jorge Canestri's investigations (Canestri, 2002) that "one of the untoward consequences of this has been a plethora of ideas and techniques described in different languages, often using the same concepts to describe entirely different ideas" (Tuckett, 2008a, p. 8).

Robert S. Wallerstein has time and again considered possible reasons that have led to a plurality of theoretical and clinical models (1988, 1990, 2002), looking for a "common ground" in psychoanalysis. His failed attempts culminate in the unsparing controversy between Wallerstein and André Green on psychoanalytic research (Green, 1996a, 1996b, see also Green, 2003; Wallerstein, 1996, 2009), as well as in the flamboyant debate on a "French-speaking view" and an "Anglo-Saxon-view" (Fonagy, 2002a) between Peter Fonagy and Roger Perron (Fonagy, 2002b; Perron, 2002, see also Perron, 2003). Perron identifies two types of "research actions": "Those where a clinical attitude prevails, and those which make use of formal and systematized procedures" (Perron, 2002, p. 3).

Facing the unsolved conundrum of the multiplicity of ways of thinking, working, and researching in psychoanalysis, Tuckett at the head of the European Psychoanalytical Federation created research groups called Working Parties. Initially, the Working Parties were intended to study firstly Theoretical Issues (*Working Party on Theoretical Issues*, WPTI); secondly, Clinical Issues (*Working Party on Clinical Issues*, WPCI); thirdly, Education (*Working Party on Education*, WPE); and finally, the Interface of psychoanalysis with other domains (*Working Party on Interface*, WPI).

The "Interface-Interview" of the Working Party on Interface and the Challenge Posed by the Wide Array of Psychotherapies

Let me start by recalling my own research experience with the research tool "Interface-Interview" within the framework of the *Working Party on Interface* (WPI) chaired by Shmuel Erlich. At that time interviewing my colleagues about their anxieties regarding the interface of psychoanalysis with the outside was quite instructive.

258

Erlich initiated and headed the short-lived EPF/FEP *Working Party on Interface* (WPI) (2000–2005) and for its task, he designed a deep interview, the "Interface-Interview." Beginning in 2003, Erlich arranged for a European-wide empirical study to be conducted by himself and his co-workers. The purpose of the semi-structured "Interface-Interview" was to explore psychoanalysts' actual exposure to and involvement with interface activities. Their attitudes towards the interface between psychoanalysis and other domains were investigated. The chosen fields of interface were psychotherapy, academia, art and culture, as well as media and politics. Some preliminary results were presented by Shmuel Erlich at the EPF/FEP in Sorrento in 2003 (Erlich, 2003). As a member of the study team, I interviewed colleagues of the society to which I belong, the Vienna Psychoanalytic Society, and I had the privilege not only to listen to the opinions of my colleagues, but also experience from a first-person perspective their emotional reactions to the questions posed by the interviewer.

In his comments on the preliminary results, Erlich reported the highest ambivalence and anxiety to be found around both psychotherapy and academia.

Regarding the interface with academia and as a sort of sequel to the EPF/FEP *Working Party on Interface* (WPI), the IPA Committee *Psychoanalysis and the University* created a forum for dialogue and the exchange of ideas. The Committee was initiated and first chaired by Ricardo Bernardi. It was later taken over by Adela Leibovich de Duarte, and finally, by Franco Borgogno,[1] but the issue of the challenge posed to psychoanalysis by the wide array of psychotherapies still remained unanswered.

The incalculable merit of the entire continuous work of the group formerly entitled *Working Party on the Specificity of Psychoanalytic Treatment Today* (WP SPTT), now named *EPF Forum The Specificity of Psychoanalytic Treatment Today*, has been to provide approaches to a comprehensive response to this question.

A seminal presentation, albeit still unpublished, of the distinguished member of this Working Party, Leopoldo Bleger, who is also a member of the IPA *Working Parties Committee*, gets to this point and maintains that specificity of psychoanalysis can neither vary according to the circumstances or history, nor be linked to a temporal condition (Bleger, 2009; see also Bleger, 2020).

Research "On" and Research "Within" Psychoanalysis

In his foreword to the second edition of *An open door review of outcome studies in psychoanalysis*, Daniel Widlöcher, at that time still president-elect, maintains that

> While clinical research remains an extremely productive tool, we must widen and complement this knowledge by other methods that are close to epidemiological studies, therapeutic trials and experimental methodology.
>
> (Widlöcher, 2001, p. V)

Later, as president of the IPA, Daniel Widlöcher differentiates a conception that considers psychoanalysis as an "object of research" and therefore generates studies "on" psychoanalysis from his own rather divergent perspective. As Widlöcher regards "psychoanalysis as a research tool," his approach allows also to conceive psychoanalytic investigations as research "within" psychoanalysis (Widlöcher, 2003, 2007).

The self-understanding of Working Parties is to investigate psychoanalysis as treatment, method, and theory by psychoanalysts. From this perspective, Serge Frisch, Leopoldo Bleger, and Evelyne Séchaud recall in the third paragraph "What kind of research in psychoanalysis?" of their article "The Specificity of Psychoanalytic Treatment Today (WPSPTT)]" (Frisch et al., 2010) this newly introduced differentiation by Daniel Widlöcher: "Research 'within' psychoanalysis is carried out by psychoanalysts qua psychoanalysts and focuses on 'psychoanalytic facts'" (Frisch et al., 2010, p. 105). The authors also refer to Jean Luc Donnet (1995), who is aware of the active presence of the unconscious within "the theory that is supposed to represent it" and to Roger Perron (1998), according to whom "theory is the major element in the constitution and construction of psychoanalytic facts" (Frisch et al., 2010, p. 106).

A *Double Vision*: Integrating Research "On" and Research "Within" Psychoanalysis

In the year 1992, Marshall Edelson, psychoanalyst and professor of psychiatry at Yale University, noted in his article "Can psychotherapy research answer this psychotherapist's questions?":

The questions a psychotherapist[2] asks as he is doing his work are questions psychotherapy research has shown little inclination to tackle. Psychotherapy research is interested, on the one hand, in big theoretical questions – in general theories of personality, pathogenesis, and psychotherapeutic process – and, on the other hand, in urgent practical questions: the outcome or efficacy of one form of psychotherapy compared to other psychotherapies, or of psychotherapy compared to other kinds of treatment.

(Edelson, 1992, pp. 118–119)

Edelson states the difficulty of translating research findings into clinical practice and has had to conclude, "The psychotherapist is interested in a particular patient and in the particular stories that patient tells or enacts" (Edelson, 1992, p. 119).

Bridging the gap between two approaches to research in psychoanalysis, Rolf Sandell terms his suggestion for a viable solution "double vision":

Double vision in research means having in mind two points of view simultaneously. One point of view involves focusing on what is generally expectable, not knowing the specifics of any particular case. . . . This is of course what nowadays is naively called "evidence" in outcome research. . . . There *are* regularities, indeed. The second point of view involves focusing on the individual differences [and using a means of synthesizing to bring some order to the individualities].

(Sandell, 2014, p. 56)

Robert S. Wallerstein joins Sandell's double vision because "this involves setting up research strategies that encompass both the generalizable and the individual . . . the formal systematic research program, and the intensive individual case study; both, not just one or the other" (Wallerstein, 2014, p. 263).

A double vision in psychoanalysis could allow both perspectives to be brought together.

On the one hand, the longstanding clinical method of our discipline established by Freud, the case study method, would neither be neglected nor eliminated from psychoanalytic research, particularly as the Working Parties take it as a starting point for elaborating their own distinctive methodologies. Additionally, a wide range of more

261

recently developed first-person empirical methodologies also could be included. On the other hand, a formal empirical and experimental research has been going from strength to strength over the past few years.

Jorge Canestri's Epistemological Frame of Reference

As an epistemological frame of reference, I would like to briefly recall some considerations of Jorge Canestri. As early as 2000, Canestri chaired the *Working Party on Theoretical Issues* (WPTI), which was devoted to investigating the meaning, use, and status of implicit theories of psychoanalysts; this means exploring their clinical practice from the *inside*, that is, the *reality* of their clinical work. The *Working Party on Theoretical Issues* also developed its own instrument for "Mapping Private Theories in Clinical Practice," theories which are mostly preconscious (Canestri, 2003, 2006, 2012).

Canestri outlines the epistemological foundation of his research while presenting the results of his Working Party in several articles and books, including *Psychoanalysis: From Practice to Theory* (2006), as well as *Putting Theory to Work: How Are Theories Actually Used in Practice?* (2012).

Even earlier, Canestri devotes a chapter, "The logic of psychoanalytic research," to this topic (Canestri, 2003) in *Pluralism and Unity? Methods of Research in Psychoanalysis*, a volume he edited with colleagues (Leuzinger-Bohleber et al., 2003). Freud's classic belief in the possibility of a junction between healing and research, a "bond between cure and research" (Freud, 1927a/1959, p. 255) [a "Junktim zwischen Heilen und Forschen" (Freud, 1927a, p. 293)], alludes to a common setting for treating patients and simultaneously carrying out research.

However, influential philosophers of science such as Hans Reichenbach and Karl Popper marked the discussion about the nature of evidence in 20th century philosophy of science by differentiating between the context of the discovery of a hypothesis, and the context of justification for validating a hypothesis (Reichenbach, 1938; Popper, 1934).

Within this framework, Freud's approach seemed to many critics to conflict with this acclaimed distinction. However, Canestri held this distinction to be unsuitable for psychoanalysis, instead preferring to embrace Imre Lakatos's (1978) recognition of an intertwining of both, the logic of discovery and the logic of justification (Canestri, 1993, 2003). Canestri has subsequently been working on a viable strategy of research for psychoanalysis (Canestri, 2003, 2012, 2015).

Some Lowest Common Denominators of Working Parties

As their lowest common denominator, the groups of the Working Parties manifest characteristics derived by Wilfred Bion's theory of "work-groups," which are structured enough in order to reduce regression and to contain its manifestations. Invoking Bion's terms, the specific group dynamics of Working Parties can be identified as including a continuous effort to contain regression; therefore, groups within Working Parties embody the ideal features of a "work-group" as conceived by Bion.

> When a group meets, it meets for a specific task, and in most human activities today co-operation has to be achieved by sophisticated means. As I have already pointed out, rules of procedure are adopted; there is usually an established administrative machinery operated by officials who are recognizable as such by the rest of the group, and so on. The capacity for co-operation on this level is great, as anybody's experience of groups will show.
>
> (Bion, 1961, p. 98)

As groups are structured in accordance with Bion's "work-groups," Working Parties are generally built on a prearranged organization (e.g., a presenter, one or two moderators, a reporter, and a group consisting of a relative stable number of participants).

In carrying on the legacy of Melanie Klein, Bion has been able to conceptualize the "group-as-a-whole" and clear the ground for further investigation of the dynamics of groups. Thus, a group can no longer be considered a simple summation of individuals, a mere collection of individual psyches or bodies, but it becomes, as Shmuel Erlich notes, referring to Bion, a "new or emergent phenomenon, obeying its own dynamics" (Erlich, 2006, p. 238). Therefore, a group is conceived as "standing in its own right and possessing characteristics, covert and overt, that transpire the individual member's psychic processes and inputs" (Erlich, 2006, p. 238). Erlich also recalls Bion's conceptions of a proto-mental level, as well as basic assumption groups, which "operate covertly at the group level, and usurp individuals to their own ends" (Erlich, 2006, p. 238).

Another common denominator of Working Parties is attention to unconscious psychophysical communication. A crucial concept is that of "mental infection" introduced by Freud in *Group psychology and the analysis of the Ego* as an "identification by means of the symptom," which he explained through an example that I elaborate next.

Freud describes the mechanism of a frequently occurring case of symptom formation. In this case, the identification leaves off the object-relation to the person who is being emulated. Freud offers the example of a pupil in a boarding school who becomes jealous because of a letter from a boy with whom she is in love:

> she reacts to it with a fit of hysterics; then some of her friends who know about it will catch the fit, as we say, by mental infection. The mechanism is that of identification based upon the possibility or desire of putting oneself in the same situation. The other girls would like to have a secret love affair too, and under the influence of a sense of guilt they also accept the suffering involved in it.
> (Freud, 1921c/1955, p. 107)

Freud proposes here that the reason her schoolmates embrace the symptom is not because they are sympathetic with the girl. On the contrary, the sympathy emerges only belatedly out of the identification. Freud adds that phenomena of infection or imitation of this kind emerge no less in groups which did not feel any pre-existing sympathy, and explains this specific process of identification in the following way:

> One ego has perceived a significant analogy with another upon one point – in our example upon openness to a similar emotion; an identification is thereupon constructed on this point, and, under the influence of the pathogenic situation, is displaced on to the symptom which the one ego has produced. The identification by means of the symptom has thus become the mark of a point of coincidence between the two egos which has to be kept repressed.
> (Freud, 1921c/1955, p. 107)

What Freud termed as "infection" has been further conceptualized by Jan Abram as "diffraction," by Haydee Faimberg as "resonance," and by the *Working Party on Microscopy of the Analytic Session* as "reverberation."

Abram's article "The inter-analytic mirror" investigates the functioning of an inter-analytic group of the *Working Party on the Specificity of Psychoanalytic Treatment Today* (WP SPTT) (Abram, 2014, 2018; see also Abram et al., 2016). It becomes apparent that the group is mirroring the analytic process of the presenting psychoanalyst. The group functions as an inter-analytic mirror in a similar way to how the psychoanalyst functions in the analytic treatment (Giampieri-Deutsch, 2018, p. 218). Abram terms this process "diffraction," which, according to Frisch, Bleger, and Séchaud, is a process occurring in an inter-analytic group: "It is the group situation that makes for this diffraction of the transference/countertransference elements amongst the participants and enables identification with these elements" (Frisch et al., 2010, p. 123).

Another common denominator of Working Parties is the emergence of parallel processes within the group (Giampieri-Deutsch, 2018, p. 218). Comparing the inter-analytic group of the *Working Party on the Specificity of Psychoanalytic Treatment Today* (WP SPTT) to the process of supervision, Frisch, Bleger, and Séchaud maintain: "In our groups, too, there is a powerful feeling of parallel processes" (Frisch et al., 2010, p. 121).

Here the authors refer to previous investigations of the triadic relationship in supervision (Fleming & Benedek, 1966; Gediman & Wolkenfeld, 1980; Innes-Smith, 1997). In these reports, the supervisees show toward their supervisors a whole string of psychic patterns that parallel the analytic processes occurring in the work they conduct with their patients (Ekstein & Wallerstein, 1958). The structural and dynamic similarities of analysis and supervision connect patient, psychoanalyst, and supervisor in a triadic relationship that allows for the emergence of parallel processes (Frisch et al., 2010, pp. 120–121).

The group's actualizations are a kind of "treatment by the group" because they allow the disavowed elements of a "treatment of the patient" to emerge. The "treatment by the group" extends and enhances the habitual understanding within the analytic relationship, leading to deeper insight into the patient for the presenting psychoanalyst (Giampieri-Deutsch, 2018, p. 219).

As stated by Frisch, Bleger, and Séchaud, members are invariably surprised upon realizing that the group can reconstruct some parts of the presented treatment, while being unable to do so for others:

That reconstruction may even be prospective, i.e., anticipating what will happen later in the course of the treatment. . . . That reconstruction is perfectly understandable, given our hypothesis that each of the participants identifies with some conscious or unconscious aspects of the patient (or of the analyst involved) and with the transference/countertransference interaction.

(Frisch et al., 2010, p. 123)

Finally, the intercorporeity discovered and studied for the first time in the psychoanalytic process within the psychoanalytic session can be experienced and investigated within the group as reported by the clinical accounts of the Working Parties. The experience of intercorporeity, the way in which psychoanalysts receive empathically the psychophysical subjectivity of their patients – including their symptoms, previously raised the interest of pioneers such as Sándor Ferenczi, Felix Deutsch, and Helene Deutsch, who explored clinically symptoms that spread from the patient to the psychoanalyst.

Taking as a starting point and inspiration the psychoanalysts of the Paris Psychosomatic School and their works, such as Pierre Marty and Michel de M'Uzan (1963), Michel Fain et al. (1964), Pierre Marty (1991), Christophe Dejours (2001), and Marilia Aisenstein (2006), different psychoanalytic approaches have further elaborated their thoughts and described this phenomenon clinically in their own case histories (Sletvold, 2014; Hartung & Steinbrecher, 2018; Birksted-Breen, 2019; Küchenhoff, 2019).

Specific Contributions of
Working Parties to Psychoanalysis

It is worth mentioning some of the plentiful and multiple achievements of Working Parties. Firstly, the Working Parties have contributed substantially to the improvement of analytic training because of the mutual exchange between training analysts working within different frames of references for training (Eitingon model, French model, Uruguayan model, etc.). This has been shown by the *Working*

Party on End of Training/Mind of the Supervisor (WP ETE), which has evolved from the formerly entitled *Working Party on Education* (WPE) (see Chapter 2 in this volume) and includes a helpful understanding of supervision by exploring what supervision is not.

The *Working Party on Microscopy of the Analytic Session* (WP MAS) (see Chapter 7 in this volume) aims to develop the analytic capacity for clinical investigation (dreaming, interpreting, validating, and theorizing) and is therefore open to candidates. This Working Party is part of the curriculum at the Institute of the Brazilian Psychoanalytic Society of São Paulo and is recognized by the Brazilian Psychoanalysis Federation (FEBRAPSI) and the Latin-American Psychoanalysis Federation (FEPAL). In addition, the "Three-Level Model for tracking change in psychoanalysis" (3-LM) – usually employed by the IPA *Committee on Clinical Observation and Testing* for its own research – has been incorporated into IPA training programs for teaching candidates how to draw up their clinical papers (see Chapter 10 in this volume).

Secondly, the *Working Party on the Specificity of Psychoanalytic Treatment Today* (WP SPTT) (see Chapter 3 in this volume) and the *Working Party on Psychosomatics* (WP P) (see Chapter 9 in this volume; see also Press et al., 2019) have shown that the intercorporeity discovered and studied for the first time within the psychoanalytic session can be experienced and investigated within the group (Giampieri-Deutsch, 2019).

Thirdly, faced with the broad range of psychotherapies, it is a tough and daunting challenge even for experienced psychoanalysts to elaborate on what distinguishes psychoanalysis from other forms of treatment. The *Working Party on the Specificity of Psychoanalytic Treatment Today* (WP SPTT) – now named *EPF Forum The Specificity of Psychoanalytic Treatment Today* – has profitably taken on this delicate task.

Fourthly, a number of Working Parties are devoted to deepening our clinical understanding, such as the *Working Party on Initiating Psychoanalysis* (WPIP) (see Chapter 5 in this volume). As Bernard Reith, current chair (2021–2023) of the IPA *Working Parties Committee*, and colleagues point out, this Working Party studies preliminary interviews that take place at the clinic to gain more insight into those dynamics which may lead to the initiation of either a psychoanalysis or a psychotherapy or, finally, may result in no treatment at all. Even though the study is heavily indebted to Bion's theoretical frame of reference, its self-understanding is to be non–theory driven and to be "a hypothesis-generating study not a hypothesis-testing study . . . based on clinical work discussed by practicing psychoanalysts, using their divergent psychoanalytic theoretical backgrounds as leverage for more precise, experience-near observation" (Reith et al., 2018, p. 4).

The breeding ground of all Working Parties committed to the study of clinical work was at its very beginning the *Working Party on Clinical Issues* (WPCI), which has also been the point of departure for Faimberg's current *Listening to Listening* (see Chapter 6 in this volume). Other Working Parties engaged in investigating clinical work are the *Working Party on Microscopy of the Analytic Session* (WP MAS) (see Chapter 7 in this volume), the *Free Clinical Groups* (FCG) (see Chapter 8 in this volume), and the IPA *Committee on Clinical Observation and Testing*, as its method is indebted to the group method of the Working Parties (see Chapter 10 in this volume).

The *Working Party on Comparative Clinical Methods* (WP CCM), now known as the *European Comparative Clinical Methods Association* (see Chapter 4 in this volume) is concerned with the enquiry into the link between theory and clinical methods. Regarding the investigation into implicit theoretical models of psychoanalysts, Tuckett remarks that the CCM method of this Working Party "can establish the facts of how someone works from their point of view; a necessary step before looking at the implicit theories they are actually using" (Tuckett, 2010, p. 11). With the two–step method, the group draws attention to the way psychoanalysts work rather than to the patient and the clinical problem. The two–step method was developed over a number of years to allow the understanding of the implicit working model of a psychoanalyst:

> It is important to distinguish these implicit models from the stereotypical and "known" official models of practice. Often these official models exist in outline form only and contain a variety of implicit models, some of which may be quite different from the official model. . . . The two-step-method steers interest away from these labels and proceeds empirically to build up an understanding of the presenting analyst's particular model.
> (Birksted-Breen et al., 2008, p. 172)

Tuckett has praised how beneficial and rewarding the permanent cooperation with Canestri's *Working Party on Theoretical Issues* (WPTI) to additionally grasp the implicit working models of a psychoanalyst has been shown to be. It is worth reminding the reader of the definition of the three-component model of theory by Canestri and colleagues in "The Map of Private (implicit, preconscious) Theories in Clinical Practice": "Theory = public theory-based thinking + private theoretical thinking + interaction of private and explicit thinking (implicit use of public theory)" (Canestri et al., 2006, p. 29; see also Canestri, 2012, p. 164).

In 2009, Charles Hanly, then president of the IPA, proposed the establishment of the IPA *Committee on Clinical Observation and Testing* (Hanly, 2014), subsequently endorsed and set up by the IPA Board. In Chapter 10 of this volume, this Committee presents its methodology and activity. This Committee, which is part of the IPA Committees for professional development, aims to explore how to make use of clinical observations to follow the process of change (or the state of the lack of change) in the patient in treatment; it intends to investigate how the observed changes have been achieved by the analyst's interventions and interpretations; it pursues the study of the process of change observed in a psychoanalysis; and finally, it makes an effort to examine on which theoretical basis interpretations and the understanding of therapeutic action of the analysts arise.

In addition, an IPA Committee finds its proper place within a volume focussed on the Working Parties because its method, the group method entitled the "Three-Level Model For Tracking Change in Psychoanalysis" (3-LM), is deeply beholden to a Working Party method (Tuckett, 2008b). Chapter 10 gives an account of Ricardo Bernardi's "Three-Level Model for Tracking Change in Psychoanalysis," a research tool for practicing psychoanalysts who are not empirical researchers. Bernardi's initial questions concerned the kinds of propositions about change that are possible for psychoanalysts and the kinds of data that should be considered by him or her for fulfilling this task (Bernardi, 2014, 2017).

Let me draw your attention to the questions of the "Three-Level Model" (3-LM) that help to understand the changes because they are derived from psychodynamic categories proposed by the Psychodynamic Diagnostic Manual (PDM, 2006) and the Operationalized Psychodynamic Diagnosis (OPD, 2008). This means that tools generally applied in empirical research could be adapted and used by clinicians for the purpose of deepening their clinical research. Clinical research and empirical research may run parallel without crossing over, but they may also become closely intertwined, as in the case of the "Three-Level Model for Tracking Change in Psychoanalysis."

Margaret Ann Fitzpatrick Hanly, chair of the IPA *Committee on Clinical Observation and Testing*, Marina Altmann de Litvan, and Ricardo Bernardi seem indeed well aware that the Three-Level Model on the one hand explores transformations in psychoanalysis by psychoanalysts, but on the other hand, that this method partly approximates to the mental health field and to its requirements for "evidence-based" practice (Fitzpatrick Hanly et al., 2021).

Along the same lines, in his "Introduction. The nature of psychoanalytic theory: Implications for psychoanalytic research," Edelson (1989) denies that "psychoanalytic research should confine itself to qualitative data" (p. 189). However, Edelson expects the chosen research instruments to be selected appropriately and to be suitable for the particular theory of psychoanalysis: "if psychoanalytic research is to make use of quantitative data in a case study, for example, its instruments for obtaining such data should be appropriate to the kind of theory it is, the kind of explanatory objectives it pursues" (Edelson, 1989, p. 189).

Nonspecific Overall Beneficial Implications of Working Parties on Psychoanalysis

In addition to the envisaged contributions of the Working Parties, a manifoldness of favourable effects on the whole psychoanalytic community needs to be kept in mind. Firstly, Working Parties continuously provide an advantageous exchange between psychoanalysts from different traditions and societies. As Paul Denis strikingly argues, "Misunderstandings between psychoanalysts from different schools and countries are not common – they are the norm" (Denis, 2008, p. 38). Moreover, he reinforces and deepens his previous statement: "Discussions between authors from different groups, when they compare theoretical elaborations, are often characterized by these ideological viewpoints and by belief systems based on a tradition that idealizes the way in which revered masters proceed" (p. 44). To counter this, the core groups of Working Parties are composed of analysts from different theoretical backgrounds and coming from different societies, initially from the EPF/FEP and then from the IPA.

Secondly, the Working Parties assured an ongoing communication between the component societies of the EPF/FEP and, later, also between the EPF/FEP and the IPA, as the activities of the Working Parties gradually extended to the IPA. In order to remedy tendencies towards mutual estrangement, the counterbalancing function of workshops and panels of the Working Parties during international psychoanalytic conferences has been to widely present the continuing activities of the Working Parties and their output, which had then undergone critical examination by other psychoanalysts and obtained a "feedback loop," as Eike Hinze, Nancy Kulish, and Marianne Robinson have formulated (see Chapter 2 in this volume). This exchange originally occurred within the EPF/FEP Conferences, then expanded outward to Regional Federations FEPAL and NAPSAC, as well as finally to the IPA Congresses.

Thirdly, in 2018 the IPA in conjunction with the Presidents of the Regional Federations marked a leap forward in quality and created the IPA *Working Parties Committee* chaired at that time by Ruggero Levy (2017–2021). This Committee overlooks the further development and integration of the Working Parties within the context of the IPA and fosters their improvement by tackling not just specific issues but rather the three general objectives of the IPA, i.e., professionalism, promotion, and participation (3 Ps). Among the inaugural activities of the IPA *Working Parties Committee* it should be emphasized that 2018 saw the start of the EPF/IPA *Working Parties Committee Joint Panels* at the 31st EPF Conference in Warsaw devoted to "The Origin of Life" under the EPF-Presidency of Jorge Canestri. The chosen topic of the first Joint Panel, "Dare we examine the origins of the psychoanalytic life of the session?," chaired by Ruggero Levy, at that time also chair (2017–2021) of the Committee and distinguished member of the *Working Party on the Specificity of Psychoanalytic Treatment Today* (WP SPTT), pursued the banding together of the clinical investigations of the Working Parties and the general theme of the conference.

Fourthly, this just bespoken integration allows psychoanalysts of the IPA coming from the different Regionals Federations to familiarize themselves at a low threshold level with both past and more recent analytic literature by peer authors belonging to other IPA societies, aside from classic and mainly quoted psychoanalytic

271

authors. Through talking about or referring to ideas from articles and books by colleagues of other societies, different or new theoretical approaches become easily accessible. All this encourages the members of the Working Parties to move onto a higher level and to achieve a greater degree of conceptualization, thus going beyond the early stage of clinical discussions. In sum, a sound knowledge or at least a better understanding of the scientific output within the IPA may contribute to a raised awareness of the productivity and liveliness of psychoanalysis in the world, and it may allow for international cooperation on overlapping topics.

Outlook: Fodor's Theory of Special Sciences

Freud's (1933a/1964) "Lecture XXXV The Question of a Weltanschauung" of his *New Introductory Lectures on Psycho-Analysis* provides a tentative taxonomy of psychoanalysis. Implicitly carrying on the legacy of his past teacher, the Darwinian and empiricist philosopher Franz Brentano (Brentano, 1874/1995, 1893/1929, p. 9),[3] Freud refused Wilhelm Dilthey's dichotomy between natural sciences and humanities and more broadly, Dilthey's German idealism; hence, Freud contends: "Strictly speaking there are only two sciences: psychology, pure and applied, and natural science" (Freud, 1933a/1964, p. 178).

As Freud doubted whether it would ever be possible to design appropriate experiments for his science, he had to conclude: "In analysis, however, we have to do without the assistance afforded to research by experiment" (Freud, 1933a/1964, p. 173).

In this lecture, Freud termed psychoanalysis "a specialist science, a branch of psychology – a depth-psychology or psychology of the unconscious" (Freud, 1933a/1964), p. 157).

In a 1995 article, Howard Shevrin creates four *dramatis personae* who embody quite different understandings of psychoanalysis. Dr. Case, one of these fictional characters, maintains "that psychoanalysis is indeed a science in its own right, with its own domain of application, phenomena, discoveries, theories, and criteria of proof" (Shevrin, 1995, p. 965). Nevertheless, Dr. Case's conception of psychoanalysis, which invokes for it the "special" status of a science *sui generis*, also entails the risk of relegating it to a *splendid isolation*.

However, alternative pathways might be followed to carry on the legacy of Freud's vision of psychoanalysis as a "specialist science."

Counterbalancing the thus far influential theory of the unity of science proposed by the Logical Empiricism of the Vienna Circle (Oppenheim & Putnam, 1958), the philosopher of mind and of science Jerry Fodor (1980, 1997) unfolded the theory of special sciences: "Reductivism is the view that all the special sciences reduce to physics" (Fodor, 1980, p. 121). Fodor shows that even though reductivism is intended to be an empirical thesis, it still aims to "play a regulative role in scientific practice" (Fodor, 1980, p. 121).

Fodor objects to this reductivist stance and upholds the scientific practice of sciences:

> Every science implies a taxonomy of the events in its universe of discourse. In particular, every science employs a descriptive vocabulary of theoretical and observation predicates, such that events fall under the laws of the science by virtue of satisfying those predicates.
>
> (Fodor, 1980, p. 123)

All those sciences which are probably not reducible to the basic physical level and which cannot derive their own theory from the theories of physics and chemistry are autonomous: "a law or a theory that figures in bona fide empirical explanations, but that is not reducible to a law or theory of physics, is ipso facto *autonomous*" (Fodor, 1997, p. 149).

At the beginning, Fodor's theory of special sciences encompassed psychology, sociology, anthropology, and economics. Fodor's positing of this theory in 1974 initiated ongoing debate, which has already lasted for decades and has resulted in the extension of the field of the special sciences. Special sciences now include biological sciences, neurophysiology, geology, astronomy, and cognitive science as well.

Endorsing both non-reductive physicalism and autonomy of special sciences, Fodor's theory would enable psychoanalysis to partake in the special sciences together with an increasing number of sciences (Giampieri-Deutsch, 2002, 2004, 2005).[4]

Notes

1 Since 2006, Erlich brought his own experiences from the *Working Party on Interface* (WPI) in his role as chairperson of the European Subcommittee of the IPA *Committee Psychoanalysis and the University*,

of which Patrizia Giampieri-Deutsch was in charge from 2012 until
its ending in 2017 due to the achievement of its objectives.

2 Even though Edelson speaks of a "psychotherapist," he means here a
"clinician," a "practising psychoanalyst."

3 During the years between 1871 and 1881 in the letters to his Romanian
friend Eduard Silberstein, Freud (1990) enthusiastically recounted his
encounter with the philosopher Franz Brentano and Freud's regular
attendance at his lessons at the University of Vienna. However, in
his writings (see Freud's *Gesammelte Werke* or *The standard edition of
the complete psychological works*), Freud did not refer to Brentano or his
theories. He mentions Brentano only once in *Jokes and their relation to
the unconscious* (Freud, 1905c/1960, pp. 31–32), as an author of riddles
(Brentano, 1879).

4 Until now, Marshall Edelson has been the only other colleague
within the scientific and psychoanalytic community to adopt
Fodor's theory of the special sciences for psychoanalysis. Edelson
once referred to Fodor's approach to object against a theoretical
reduction of psychoanalysis by neuroscience. Edelson obviously did
not reject the idea that mental states are embodied or that they
have neuropsychological correlates, but he strongly disfavoured a
theoretical reduction of psychoanalysis. This would be indeed a difficult, daunting task, because in a theoretical reduction, "we shall
be able to demonstrate that the concepts of a psychology of mind
correspond to concepts of neuroscience, and that the explanatory
generalizations of a psychology of mind can be logically derived
from explanatory generalizations of neuroscience" (Edelson, 1986,
p. 480). Meanwhile, after all these years, neuroscience too claims
the autonomy of a special science.

5 The chronological order of Freud's writings (showed using let-
ters of the alphabet) is based upon the volume Meyer-Palmedo, I.,
& Fichtner, G. (Eds.) (1989). *Freud-Bibliographie mit Werkkonkordanz*
[Freud-bibliography and concordance of his publications] (pp. 15–90).
Frankfurt am Main: Fischer.

Bibliography[5]

Abram, J. (2014). Le miroir inter-analytique: Son rôle dans la reconnaissance des traumas trans-générationnels désavoués [The inter-analytic
mirror: Its role in recognising disavowed trauma]. *Revue Française de
Psychanalyse*, 78 (2), 405–416.

Abram, J. (2018). The inter-analytic mirror. *Psychoanalysis in Europe:
Bulletin of the European Psychoanalytical Federation (EPF)*, 72,
203–209.

Abram, J., Bleger, L., & Valon, P. (2016). The specificity of psychoanalytic treatment today: A Working Party of the EPF [Paper presentation] Annual Research Lecture to the BPaS, *Bulletin of the British Psychoanalytic Society*. (Original work published 2015).

Aisenstein, M. (2006). The indissociable unity of psyche and soma: A view from the Paris psychosomatic school. *International Journal of Psychoanalysis*, *87* (3), 667–680.

Bernardi, R. (2014). The Three-Level-Model (3-LM) for observing patient transformations. In M. Altmann de Litvan (Ed.), *Time for change: Tracking transformations in psychoanalysis – The Three-Level Model* (pp. 3–34). Karnac Books.

Bernardi, R. (2017). A common ground in clinical discussion groups: Intersubjective resonance and implicit operational theories. *International Journal of Psychoanalysis*, *98* (5), 1291–1309.

Bion, W. R. (1961). *Experiences in groups and other papers*. Tavistock Publications Limited.

Birksted-Breen, D. (2019). Pathways of the unconscious: When the body is the receiver/instrument. *International Journal of Psychoanalysis*, *100* (6), 1117–1133.

Birksted-Breen, D., Ferro, A., & Mariotti, P. (2008). Work in progress: Using the two-step method. In D. Tuckett, R. Basile, D. Birksted-Breen, T. Böhm, P. Denis, A. Ferro, H. Hinz, A. Jemsted, P. Mariotti, & J. Schubert (Eds.), *Psychoanalysis comparable and incomparable: The evolution of a method to describe and compare psychoanalytic approaches* (pp. 167–207). The New Library of Psychoanalysis, Routledge.

Bleger, L. (2009). Présentation à l'Association Psychanalytique de France (APF) en Mai 2009 [Presentation at the French Psychoanalytical Association in Mai 2009] [Paper presentation] French Psychoanalytical Association.

Bleger, L. (2020). L'idéal et le transfert dans la formation des psychanalystes [The ideal and the transference in the forming of psychoanalysts]. *Revue Française de Psychanalyse*, *84* (1), 177–184.

Brentano, F. (1879). *Aegnimatias [Riddles]*. C. Gerold Sohn.

Brentano, F. (1929). Über die Zukunft der Philosophie [On the future of philosophy]. In *Über die Zukunft der Philosophie [On the future of philosophy]* (pp. 7–81). Meiner Verlag. (Original work published 1893).

Brentano, F. (1995). *Psychology from an empirical standpoint*, L. L. McAlister (Ed.). Routledge. (Original work published 1874).

Canestri, J. (1993). The logic of Freudian research. In D. Meghnagi (Ed.), *Freud and Judaism* (pp. 117–129). Karnac Books.

Canestri, J. (2002). Projective identification. The fate of the concept in Italy and Spain. *Psychoanalysis in Europe: European Psychoanalytical Federation Bulletin*, *56*, 130–139.

Canestri, J. (2003). The logic of psychoanalytic research. In M. Leuzinger-Bohleber, A. U. Dreher, & J. Canestri (Eds.), *Pluralism and unity? Methods of research in psychoanalysis* (pp. 137–148). International Psychoanalysis Library.

Canestri, J. (Ed.) (2006). *Psychoanalysis: From practice to theory.* Wiley Blackwell.

Canestri, J. (Ed.) (2012). *Putting theory to work: How are theories actually used in practice?* Karnac Books.

Canestri, J. (2015). The case for neuropsychoanalysis. *International Journal of Psychoanalysis, 96* (6), 1575–1584.

Canestri, J., Bohleber, W., Denis, P., & Fonagy, P. (2006). The map of private (implicit, preconscious) theories in clinical practice. In J. Canestri (Ed.), *Psychoanalysis: From practice to theory* (pp. 29–43). Wiley Blackwell.

Cooper, A. (2003). Commentary on "Psychoanalytic discourse at the turn of our century": A plea for a measure of humanity. *Journal of the American Psychoanalytic Association, 51*, 108–114.

Denis, P. (2008). In praise of empiricism. In D. Tuckett, R. Basile, D. Birksted-Breen, T. Böhm, P. Denis, A. Ferro, H. Hinz, A. Jemsted, P. Mariotti, & J. Schubert (Eds.), *Psychoanalysis comparable and incomparable: The evolution of a method to describe and compare psychoanalytic approaches* (pp. 38–49). The New Library of Psychoanalysis, Routledge.

Dejours, C. (2018). *Le corps, d'abord – Corps biologique, corps érotique et sens moral [The body, first and foremost – biological body, erotic body, and moral sense].* Petite Bibliothèque Payot No. 476. (Original work published 2001).

Donnet, J. L. (1995). L'opération Méta [The operation Meta]. In *Le divan bien tempéré [The well-tempered couch].* Presse Universitaire de France.

Edelson, M. (1986). The convergence of psychoanalysis and neuroscience: Illusion and reality. *Contemporary Psychoanalysis, 22*, 479–519.

Edelson, M. (1989). Introduction: The nature of psychoanalytic theory: Implications for psychoanalytic research. *Psychoanalytic Inquiry, 9* (2), 169–192.

Edelson, M. (1992). Can psychotherapy research answer this psychotherapist's questions? *Contemporary Psychoanalysis, 28*, 118–151.

Ekstein, R., & Wallerstein, R. S. (1958). *The teaching and learning of psychotherapy.* Basic Books.

Erlich, H. S. (2003). Relating to the outside: Presentation of preliminary results of the Working Party on Interface [Paper presentation] Conference of European Psychoanalytical Federation (EPF), Sorrento, Italy.

Erlich, H. S. (2006). Der Mann Freud: A contemporary perspective on his and our Jewish and psychoanalytic identity. In R. Ginsburg,

& I. Pardes (Eds.), *New perspectives on Freud's "Moses and Monotheism"* (pp. 235–244). Max Niemeyer Verlag.

Fain, M., David, C., & Marty, P. (1964). Perspective psychosomatique sur la fonction des fantasmes [A psychosomatic perspective on the function of fantasies]. *Revue Française de Psychanalyse, 28*, 609–622.

Fitzpatrick Hanly, M. A., Altmann de Litvan, M., & Bernardi, R. (Eds.) (2021). *Change through time in psychoanalysis, transformations and interventions: The Three-Level Model.* Routledge.

Fleming, J., & Benedek, T. (1966). *Psychoanalytic supervision.* Grune & Stratton.

Fodor, J. (1980). Special sciences, or the disunity of science as a working hypothesis. In N. Block (Ed.), *Readings in philosophy of psychology* (Vol. 1, pp. 120–133). Harvard University Press. (Original work published 1974).

Fodor, J. (1997). Special sciences: Still autonomous after all these years. *Noûs, 31*, 149–163.

Fonagy, P. (Ed.) (2002a). *An open door review of outcome studies in psychoanalysis.* International Psychoanalytical Association.

Fonagy, P. (2002b). Epistemological and methodological background: Part 2-B: Reflections on psychoanalytic research problems – An AngloSaxon view. In P. Fonagy (Ed.), *An open door review of outcome studies in psychoanalysis* (pp. 10–29). International Psychoanalytical Association.

Freud, S. (1927a) Nachwort zur Frage der Laienanalyse. Unterredungen mit einem Unparteiischen [Postscript to The question of lay analysis: Conversations with an impartial person]. In A. Freud (Ed.), *Gesammelte Werke* (Vol. 14, pp. 287–296). Fischer.

Freud, S. (1955). Group psychology and the analysis of the ego. In J. Strachey (Ed. & Trans.), *The standard edition of the complete psychological works of Sigmund Freud* (Vol. 18, pp. 65–144). Hogarth Press. (Original work published 1921c).

Freud, S. (1959). Postscript to the question of lay analysis: Conversations with an impartial person. In J. Strachey (Ed. & Trans.), *The standard edition of the complete psychological works of Sigmund Freud* (Vol. 20, pp. 251–258). Hogarth Press. (Original work published 1927a).

Freud, S. (1960). Jokes and their relation to the unconscious. In J. Strachey (Ed. & Trans.), *The standard edition of the complete psychological works of Sigmund Freud* (Vol. 8). Hogarth Press. (Original work published 1905c).

Freud, S. (1964). Lecture XXXV the question of a Weltanschauung: New introductory lectures on psycho–analysis. In J. Strachey (Ed. & Trans.), *The standard edition of the complete psychological works of Sigmund Freud* (Vol. 22, pp. 157–182). Hogarth Press. (Original work published 1933a).

Freud, S. (1990). *The letters of Sigmund Freud to Eduard Silberstein 1871–1881*, W. Boehlich (Ed.), A. J. Pomerans (Trans.). The Belknap Press of Harvard University Press.

Frisch, S., Bleger, L., & Séchaud, E. (2010). Die Spezifität psychoanalytischer Behandlungen heute [The Specificity of Psychoanalytic Treatment Today (WPSPTT)]. *Psychoanalyse in Europa: Bulletin der Europäischen Psychoanalytischen Föderation (EPF)*, *64* (Supplement), 98–127.

Gediman, H., & Wolkenfeld, F. (1980). The parallelism phenomenon in psychoanalysis and supervision: Its reconsideration as a triadic system. *Psychoanalytic Quarterly, 49*, 234–255.

Giampieri-Deutsch, P. (Ed.) (2002). *Psychoanalyse im Dialog der Wissenschaften. Europäische Perspektiven [Psychoanalysis in a dialogue among sciences. European perspectives]* (Vol. 1). Kohlhammer.

Giampieri-Deutsch, P. (Ed.) (2004). *Psychoanalyse im Dialog der Wissenschaften: Angloamerikanische Perspektiven [Psychoanalysis in a dialogue among sciences. Anglo-American perspectives]* (Vol. 2). Kohlhammer.

Giampieri-Deutsch, P. (Ed.) (2005). *Psychoanalysis as an empirical, interdisciplinary science. Collected papers on contemporary psychoanalytic research.* Austrian Academy of Sciences Press.

Giampieri-Deutsch, P. (2018). Dare we examine the origins of the psychoanalytic life of the session? Discussion: Two examples of research "within" psychoanalysis. *Psychoanalyse in Europe: Bulletin of the European Psychoanalytical Federation (EPF)*, *72*, 215–222.

Giampieri-Deutsch, P. (2019). The body in inter-analytic investigation: Object and subject, source and resource. Discussion of L. Michel's "Body and specificity: Bodily expressions in the inter-analytic group" & M. Perris-Myttas' "The Working Party on psychosomatics: A journey of exploration". [Panel presentation]. 32nd Conference of the European Psychoanalytical Federation (EPF): Body, EPF/IPA Working Parties Committee Joint Panel, Madrid, Spain.

Green, A. (1996a). What kind of research for psychoanalysis? *Newsletter of the IPA*, 5, 10–14.

Green, A. (1996b). Response to Robert S. Wallerstein. *Newsletter of the IPA, 5*, 18–21.

Green, A. (2003). The pluralism of sciences and psychoanalytic thinking. In M. Leuzinger-Bohleber, A. U. Dreher, & J. Canestri (Eds.), *Pluralism and unity? Methods of research in psychoanalysis* (pp. 26–44). International Psychoanalysis Library.

Hanly, C. (2014). Foreword. In M. Altmann (Ed.), *Time for change: Tracking transformations in psychoanalysis – The Three-Level Model* (pp. ix – xxiv). Karnac Books.

Innes-Smith, J. (1997). Être ou ne pas être . . . analyste [To be or not to be . . . an analyst]. *Psychanalyse in Europe: Bulletin of the Fédération Européenne de Psychanalyse, 48*, 95–107.

Hartung, T., & Steinbrecher, M. (2018). From somatic pain to psychic pain: The body in the psychoanalytic field. *International Journal of Psychoanalysis, 99* (1), 159–180.

Küchenhoff, J. (2019). Intercorporeity and body language: The semiotics of mental suffering expressed through the body. *International Journal of Psychoanalysis, 100* (4), 769–791.

Lakatos, I. (1978). *Proofs and refutations: The logic of mathematical discovery.* Cambridge University Press.

Leuzinger-Bohleber, M., Dreher, A. U., & Canestri, J. (Eds.) (2003). *Pluralism and unity? Methods of research in psychoanalysis.* International Psychoanalysis Library.

Marty, M., & de M'Uzan, M. (1963). La pensée opératoire [The operational thinking]. *Revue Française de Psychanalyse, 27*, 345–355.

Marty, P. (1991). *Mentalisation et psychosomatique [Mentalization and psychosomatics].* Laboratoire Delagrange.

Michels, R. (2007). Optimal education requires an academic context: Commentary on Wallerstein. *Journal of the American Psychoanalytic Association, 55*, 985–989.

OPD Task Force (2008). *Operationalized psychodynamic diagnosis manual of diagnosis and treatment planning.* Hogrefe and Huber.

Oppenheim, P., & Putnam, H. (1958). Unity of science as a working hypothesis. In H. Feigl, M. Scriven, & G. Maxwell (Eds.), *Minnesota studies in the philosophy of science* (Vol. 2, pp. 3–36). University of Minnesota Press.

PDM (2006). *Psychodynamic diagnostic manual.* Alliance of Psychoanalytic Organizations.

Perron, R. (1998). La recherche en psychanalyse et l'Association Psychanalytique Internationale [Research in psychoanalysis and the International Psychoanalytical Association]. *Bulletin de la Société Psychanalytique de Paris, 50*, 39–51.

Perron, R. (2002). Epistemological and methodological background: Part 2-A: Reflections on psychoanalytic research problems – A French-speaking view. In P. Fonagy (Ed.), *An open door review of outcome studies in psychoanalysis* (pp. 3–9). International Psychoanalytical Association.

Perron, R. (2003). What are we looking for? How? In M. Leuzinger-Bohleber, A. U. Dreher, & J. Canestri (Eds.), *Pluralism and unity? Methods of research in psychoanalysis* (pp. 97–108). International Psychoanalysis Library.

Popper, K. R. (1934). *Logik der Forschung [The logic of scientific discovery]*. Mohr.

Press, J., Bobos, F., Frommer, J., Perris-Myttas, M., Schmid-Gloor, E., de Senarclens, B., Seulin, C., Solano, L., Temple, N., & Humble, C. (2019). *Experiencing the body: A psychoanalytic dialogue on psychosomatics*. The New Library of Psychoanalysis, Routledge.

Reichenbach, H. (1938). *Experience and prediction: An analysis of the foundations and the structure of knowledge*. The University of Chicago Press.

Reith, B., Moller, M., Boots, J., Crick, P., Gibeault, A., Jaffee, R., Langerlof, S., & Vermote, R. (2018). *Beginning analysis: On the processes of initiating psychoanalysis*. The New Library of Psychoanalysis, Routledge.

Sandell, R. (2014). On the value of double vision. *Contemporary Psychoanalysis, 50* (1–2), 43–57.

Shevrin, H. (1995). Is psychoanalysis one science, two sciences, or no science at all? A discourse among friendly antagonists. *Journal of the American Psychoanalytic Association, 43*, 963–986.

Sletvold, J. (2014). *The embodied analyst – from Freud and Reich to relationality*. Routledge.

Tuckett, D. (2008a). On difference, discussing differences and comparison: An introduction. In D. Tuckett, R. Basile, D. Birksted-Breen, T. Böhm, P. Denis, A. Ferro, H. Hinz, A. Jemstedt, P. Mariotti, & J. Schubert (Eds.), *Psychoanalysis comparable and incomparable: The evolution of a method to describe and compare psychoanalytic approaches* (pp. 5–37). The New Library of Psychoanalysis, Routledge.

Tuckett, D. (2008b). Reflection and evolution: Developing the Two-Step Method. In D. Tuckett, R. Basile, D. Birksted-Breen, T. Böhm, P. Denis, A. Ferro, H. Hinz, A. Jemstedt, P. Mariotti, & J. Schubert (Eds.), *Psychoanalysis comparable and incomparable: The evolution of a method to describe and compare psychoanalytic approaches* (pp. 132–166). The New Library of Psychoanalysis, Routledge.

Tuckett, D. (2010). Wie arbeiten Psychoanalytiker? Die Arbeit der EPF-Arbeitsgruppe über vergleichende klinische Methoden, 2003–2009 [How do psychoanalysts work? The work of the EPF Working Party on comparative clinical methods 2003–2009]. *Psychoanalyse in Europa: Bulletin der Europäischen Psychoanalytischen Föderation, 64* (Supplement), 5–35.

Tuckett, D., Basile, R., Birksted-Breen, D., Böhm, T., Denis, P., Ferro, A., Hinz, H., Jemstedt, A., Mariotti, P., & Schubert, J. (Eds.) (2008). *Psychoanalysis comparable and incomparable: The evolution of a method to describe and compare psychoanalytic approaches*. The New Library of Psychoanalysis, Routledge.

Wallerstein, R. S. (1988). One psychoanalysis or many? *International Journal of Psychoanalysis, 69* (1), 5–21.

Wallerstein, R. S. (1990). Psychoanalysis: The common ground. *International Journal of Psychoanalysis, 71* (1), 3–20.

Wallerstein, R. S. (1996). Psychoanalytic research: Where do we disagree? *Newsletter of the IPA, 5,* 15–17.

Wallerstein, R. S. (2002). The trajectory of psychoanalysis: A prognostication. *International Journal of Psychoanalysis, 83* (6), 1247–1267.

Wallerstein, R. S. (2009). What kind of research in psychoanalytic science? *International Journal of Psychoanalysis, 90* (1), 109–133.

Wallerstein, R. S. (2014). Psychoanalytic therapy research: A commentary. In R. Coleman Curtis (Ed.), *Contemporary Psychoanalysis: Special Section: Systematic Research on Psychoanalytic Treatment, 50* (1–2), 259–269.

Widlöcher, D. (2001). Preface. In P. Fonagy (Ed.), *An open door review of outcome studies in psychoanalysis (2002)* (p. V). International Psychoanalytical Association.

Widlöcher, D. (2003). Foreword. In M. Leuzinger-Bohleber, A. U. Dreher, & J. Canestri (Eds.), *Pluralism and unity? Methods of research in psychoanalysis* (pp. XIX–XXIV). International Psychoanalysis Library.

Widlöcher, D. (2007). La recherche: pour qui et pour quel débat [Research: For whom and for what debate]. In M. Emmanuelli, & R. Perron, (Eds.), *La recherche en psychanalyse [The research in psychoanalysis]* (pp. 39–52). Presse Universitaire de France.

Index

Note: Page numbers followed by "n" with numbers refer to notes.

Faimberg, H. 14, 143–156, 157n3, 265, 268; *see also Listening to listening* (Faimberg)
Fain, M. 266
fear 69, 74, 96, 101–108, 184–185, 207–209
feeling 93–97, 101–105, 189–190, 204–207, 229–230
FEP 150–152, 259, 271
Ferenczi, S. 208, 266
Ferro, A. 79, 219
first zone of transition 202–203
Fodor, J. 273
folie à deux 217
Fonagy, P. 258
forbidden love 56
free association 70
Free Clinical Groups (FCG) method 176, 181–186; development of 190–192; emotionality 179–180; group discussion 186–190; opening scenes 180–181; prisma effect, options of interpretation, and the episode 176–179
Freud, S. 1–2, 65–66, 202, 204, 262–265, 272, 274n3
Frisch, S. 260, 266

Gabbard, G. 95
Gattig, E. 176
Gediman, H. K. 40
Geverif, R. 12
Giampieri-Deutsch, P. 29
Glover, B. 112, 122
Glover, W. 112
Green, A. 202–204, 210, 220, 258
Grounded Theory 10
group-as-a-whole 263
group discussion 186–190
Gullestad, S. E. 227

habitual phrases 234
Haesler, L. 44

Hanly, C. 223, 269
Hanly, F. 223–224, 247
Hanly, M. A. F. 223, 270
Hinze, E. 36–37, 271
hope 8, 12, 28, 164, 201
hypothesis 111, 133–135, 266, 268
hypothetical interpretations 165–166

implicit theories 167–168
impulse 119, 185, 201–202, 217, 245
infantile sexual fantasies 5, 75–78
infections 46–47, 265
inner reality 181–182
inseparable bond 20
institution: atmosphere of 43; containment function of 46–47
institutional impingement 42–43; and identification with a patient 50–51; and parallel process 48–49, 51–53; and transference 49–50
inter-analytic group 6, 79, 265
inter-clinical exchange group 79
Interface-Interview 258–259
internal work 141–142
International Psychoanalytical Association (IPA) 13–16, 62, 67, 269–272
interpersonal relationship 244, 252
Interpretation of Dreams (Freud) 201–202, 210, 212
intimacy 50, 105, 107–108, 232
intrapsychic conflicts 245, 252–253
isomorphism 76

Junkers, G. 36

Kächele, H. 228
Kaës, R. 10, 79
Klein, M. 263

For Product Safety Concerns and Information please contact our EU
representative GPSR@taylorandfrancis.com
Taylor & Francis Verlag GmbH, Kaufingerstraße 24, 80331 München, Germany

9 781032 656281